"Holland and Hawks are to be commended for this concise and accessible review of a range of empirically supported Mindfulness and Acceptance and Commitment Therapy practices. Especially relevant for the busy school mental health professional, I particularly appreciated its use of a Multi-Tiered System of Support (MTSS) perspective. Virtually all educators will find something relevant to their practice in this book's school-wide, classroom, small group, and individual approaches (which include a range of forms and implementation resources)."

Stephen E. Brock, *PhD, NCSP, LEP*
Professor & School Psychology Program Coordinator, California State University, Sacramento

"How do we calm our minds when our thoughts act like tigers? This book is a road map for school-based practitioners interested in integrating mindfulness and ACT practices into their MTSS model. Holland and Hawks have created a practical guide that includes the fundamentals of ACT and mindfulness practices, giving detailed real-world examples and easy-to-use strategies that can be implemented in the school system. This is an extraordinary resource for those in education."

Danielle McIntyre, *EdS*
School Psychologist & RYT200 Yoga Instructor, Santa Rosa County School District

"Given the mental health crisis amongst youth, there is an urgent need to expand school-based mental health services and support. This book provides a practical and comprehensive guide to implement evidence-based interventions to support <u>all</u> students. This book fills a critical need and is a 'must have' for all teachers and school-based practitioners."

McKenzie Courtney, *EdS*
School Psychologist & Licensed Educational Psychologist, Buckeye Union School District

Mindfulness and Acceptance and Commitment Practices in the School Setting

This book offers specific, easy-to-implement mindfulness and acceptance and commitment therapy (ACT) tools for practitioners to use in schools at an individual, group, or classroom-wide level.

With the increased focus on the emotional and behavioral health of children in the schools, there is a dearth of practical books that specifically address the use of ACT techniques in the school setting. Geared toward the practitioner and how they work with students, teachers, parents, and classrooms, this book introduces a contemporary approach to targeted intervention and discusses how these services can be provided using an MTSS model. These interventions have numerous benefits including increasing attention capacity, compassion, emotional regulation, and self-calming abilities, in addition to use as an intervention for anxiety, depression, and trauma related symptoms.

Graduate students and practitioners who work with children and adolescents such as school psychologists, child and adolescent clinical psychologists, and school counselors will find this book to be a novel resource of interventions for children in grades K–12, along with tools to support parents and teachers.

Melissa L. Holland, PhD is a professor in the School Psychology Program at California State University, Sacramento and is a practicing clinical psychologist.

Jessica L. Hawks, PhD is a clinical child and adolescent psychologist, an associate professor at the University of Colorado, and the Clinical Director of the Pediatric Mental Health Institute, Children's Hospital Colorado.

Mindfulness and Acceptance and Commitment Practices in the School Setting

Practical Interventions for Children and Adolescents

Melissa L. Holland
and Jessica L. Hawks

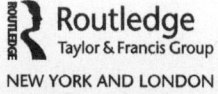
Routledge
Taylor & Francis Group

NEW YORK AND LONDON

Cover image: Getty Images

First published 2023
by Routledge
605 Third Avenue, New York, NY 10158

and by Routledge
4 Park Square, Milton Park, Abingdon, Oxon, OX14 4RN

Routledge is an imprint of the Taylor & Francis Group, an informa business

© 2023 Melissa L. Holland and Jessica L. Hawks

The right of Melissa L. Holland and Jessica L. Hawks to be identified as authors of this work has been asserted in accordance with sections 77 and 78 of the Copyright, Designs and Patents Act 1988.

ISBN: 978-1-032-33083-9 (hbk)
ISBN: 978-1-032-33082-2 (pbk)
ISBN: 978-1-003-31810-1 (ebk)

DOI: 10.4324/9781003318101

Typeset in NewBaskerville
by Apex CoVantage, LLC

I dedicate this book to my children, Sophia and Colette, and to all those working in the schools to better the mental health of the children they serve.

– Melissa L. Holland, PhD

I dedicate this book to my family – Brianna, Aiden, and Alexander.

– Jessica L. Hawks, PhD

Contents

About the Authors

Melissa L. Holland, PhD, is a professor of School Psychology at the California State University, Sacramento (CSUS) and has a private practice specializing in work with children, adolescents, and their families. She is both a licensed clinical psychologist and a certified school psychologist. Her publications and presentations focus on the emotional health of children and burnout and compassion fatigue for providers in the helping professions. She acts as a consultant in schools on the topic of social emotional learning and the use of mindfulness, cognitive, and behavioral strategies with students. She has worked extensively in the area of trauma and mental health in the schools, including clinical work, trainings for school districts, and research-related activities. She is also the mother of two daughters, Sophia and Colette.

Jessica L. Hawks, PhD, is a clinical child and adolescent psychologist and the clinical director of the Pediatric Mental Health Institute, Children's Hospital Colorado. She is also an associate professor in the Department of Psychiatry, School of Medicine, at the University of Colorado. Dr. Hawks' clinical expertise is in working with youth with behavioral difficulties and/or chronic irritability and their parents. Her research focuses on innovative clinical program development and dissemination efforts aimed at bringing a transdiagnostic approach to pediatric mental health assessment and treatment services. Dr. Hawks is routinely invited to interview for state and national media outlets, as well as provide community lectures, on pediatric mental health. Her professional presentations and publications focus on transdiagnostic clinical interventions for youth and families. She is married and has two sons, Aiden and Alexander.

Preface

Throughout this book, several key terms and pronouns will be utilized. Specifically, the terms "practitioner," "youth," and "parent" will be used, along with non-gendered language to refer to individuals or groups. The term "practitioner" is meant to describe any professional who provides mental health supports to youth. The term "youth" will be used to reference individuals from early childhood through adolescence. Alterations in the use of techniques for different age levels will be specified when necessary (e.g., some approaches may not be appropriate for very young children, or modifications will be offered). The term "parent" will be used to encompass all primary caregivers, regardless of biological relation. Finally, non-gendered language will be used throughout the text, with the pronouns of they/them/their utilized, as opposed to he/him/his or she/her/hers, as is consistent with inclusive language. Case examples will specify preferred pronouns.

Acknowledgments

We want to thank Routledge/Taylor & Francis Group for their support and assistance in the process of bringing this book to fruition. Thank you to Sophia Beckette, our illustrator for this book. We also appreciate the support of our universities, colleagues, and students during this journey of writing this book. We hope this book will be useful for all those who work with youth in the school setting.

1   Introduction to Mindfulness and ACT Practices

Roadmap to Chapter 1:
This chapter defines mindfulness and ACT practices and explains why you should use these in the schools.

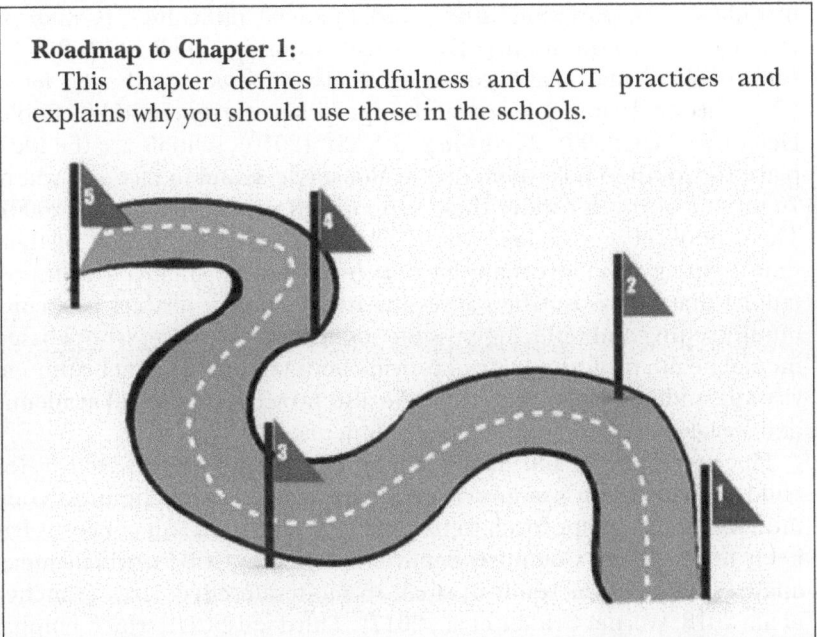

Promotion of childhood mental health is critical to the lifelong well-being of our youth and includes ensuring they meet developmental milestones, develop appropriate social skills, and learn how to effectively cope with adversity. Without such skills, youth are at risk for a variety of negative outcomes including academic difficulties, delinquency, poorer physical health, and relational problems (National Association of School Psychologists [NASP], 2016).

Developmental research has concluded that approximately 50% of all psychiatric illnesses have an onset before the age of 14 and that the mean onset of symptoms precedes the full diagnosis by approximately two years (National Institute of Medicine, 2009). Left untreated, it has been

DOI: 10.4324/9781003318101-1

estimated that approximately 50% of young children who show early signs of internalizing concerns, such as anxiety (Carballo et al., 2010; Slemming et al., 2010) or externalizing concerns, such as attentional deficits or conduct problems (Hong et al., 2015;Riddle et al., 2013), will continue to experience these problems over time. Thus, prevention and early intervention services are crucial to thwarting later, more serious, mental health challenges for youth.

The Centers for Disease Control and Prevention (CDC, 2013) have estimated that approximately one in five youth experience a mental health disorder in any given year. Despite the rising numbers of youth mental health concerns, significant barriers exist to accessing necessary treatment including mental health stigma, a shortage of mental health providers, transportation issues, and financial difficulties (California Department of Education [CDE], 2020). Consequentially, only 20% of youth with mental health concerns receive treatment and even fewer (7%) receive evidence-based and appropriate treatment (U.S. Public Health Service, 2000). According to NASP (2016), schools are the ideal place for youth to receive mental health services, and in fact, it is where 70 to 80% of youth receive these supports (Rones & Hoagwood, 2000). The school setting is where youth spend a significant portion of their time, helping to remove many barriers (e.g., cultural, financial, transportation) that may exist when accessing mental health services in a community setting and reducing possible stigma. Furthermore, school-based mental health professionals can provide both targeted mental health services to students with concerns, while also providing universal academic and social-emotional supports to all students.

The development and dissemination of evidence-based practices for child mental health has grown rapidly in recent years. The most common school-based approach to treatment of mental health concerns has been informed by Cognitive Behavioral Therapy (CBT), which meta-analyses have shown result in small to moderate effect sizes (Sanchez et al., 2018; Werner-Seidler et al., 2017). Third-wave CBT, which emphasizes the use of mindfulness and ACT based practices, has recently emerged as an alternative approach in addressing youth mental health concerns. Mindfulness and ACT practices target underlying psychological processes, rather than specific symptoms, resulting in a more flexible and universally applicable approach. While there is robust literature available regarding mindfulness-based practices with children, few publications have focused on the addition of acceptance and commitment-based practices in the school setting. Given that use of ACT practices has been shown to have a positive additive effect when used in conjunction with mindfulness (Chin et al., 2019), increased focus must be placed on the integration of these approaches.

The purpose of this book is to describe how school-based professionals can use mindfulness and ACT practices in the school setting to support the mental health needs of the students they serve. We will cover the use of mindfulness and ACT practices across the multi-tiered system of support (MTSS) model including universal and school-wide supports (Tier 1), small group work (Tier 2), and individualized, intensive intervention (Tier 3).

The Multi-Tiered System of Supports

Within the MTSS, three levels or tiers of support can be given, depending on the youth's level of need. Most children (about 80%) will be functioning as expected, needing no formal social-emotional-behavioral intervention. At the Tier 1 level, children receive services in the general classroom, with class-wide or schoolwide prevention and early intervention services. These universal, core interventions target the whole student population (Salerno, 2016). Common Tier 1 interventions include the general, classroom-wide social and emotional curriculum or positive behavior intervention support practices in the schools that apply to all students. Youth at risk for social, emotional, or behavioral problems receive services at the Tier 2 level of support. Approximately 15% of children are at this level and receive more targeted prevention and early intervention, often in small groups. Types of Tier 2 intervention include small, pull-out groups focusing on a particular skill, area of concern, or peer tutoring. At the Tier 3 level, children are at the highest risk for problems. The 5% of children at this level typically receive more individualized and intensive interventions, such as one-on-one counseling (Holland et al., 2017). One of the many benefits of using mindfulness and acceptance-based techniques in the school setting is that they are quite flexible, and thus, can be effectively applied at the Tier 1, 2, or 3 levels.

The remainder of this chapter will describe the concepts of mindfulness and ACT. We will also outline the benefits of using these practices in a school setting when addressing the mental health needs of youth. We will conclude with an overview of the rest of the book.

What Is Mindfulness?

Mindfulness has been defined in a variety of ways. Definitions of mindfulness are often subject to the practitioner's or researcher's own understanding of the experience (Albrecht et al., 2012). One common definition is that mindfulness is a way of attending to the present moment in a reflective fashion, without judgment or comparisons (Rechtschaffen, 2016). Kabat-Zinn's (1994, p. 4) popular definition of mindfulness is frequently found throughout the literature – "paying attention in a particular way: on purpose, in the present moment and non-judgmentally." Shapiro and colleagues (2006), have said that Kabat-Zinn's definition involves three axioms: intention, attention, and attitude.

The first axiom, intention, is seen as integral to mindfulness practice. Your vision for how mindfulness will assist or affect your life can be instrumental in determining the outcome of the practice (Shapiro et al., 2006). For example, a highly stressed person may begin a mindfulness practice to reduce their high blood pressure. As they continue using mindfulness, that person may then develop an additional intention of becoming less reactive toward others.

Attention, the second axiom, involves the individual paying attention in the moment to both their internal and external experience in a sustained and regulated way. Attention is considered an essential element in the healing process (Shapiro et al., 2006): that which we focus on expands and can be acknowledged, repeated, and reinforced (Tolle, 1999). For example, the more we use our senses to pay attention to what is around us, the less we are attending to past or future oriented thoughts, which can increase feelings of depression or anxiety. Such a focus on present moment sensations could be beneficial for our mental well-being.

Finally, attitude, the third axiom, concerns the qualities that users bring to their mindfulness practice. This is what Kabat-Zinn (1994) means by "in a particular way." For example, individuals could observe their life with a cold and distant attitude or, conversely, pay attention from a state of open-heartedness, peace, and compassion (Shapiro et al., 2006). This latter way of attending has been called "heartfulness" and is seen as a critical part of mindful living in many practices (Daugherty, 2014). Heartfulness has been defined as having a warm, heartfelt relationship with whatever is happening in your experience, internal or external; it is also the capacity to regard yourself, others, and the world with a sense of empathy and kindness (Mindful Schools, 2015a). All three axioms as defined by Shapiro et al. (2006) are typically included in mindfulness interventions and programs.

One benefit of mindfulness is that it can change our attachment and relationship to our thoughts. Having thoughts of varied emotional valence is completely normal and mindfulness does not aim to get rid of thoughts. Rather, the aim is to see thoughts for what they really are. Thoughts are not facts; they are simply events in the brain. In this way, thoughts are neither "good" nor "bad," they are simply information. When we get lost in the content of our thoughts, we stop being in the present. Mindfulness is about learning to realize when we're caught up in thoughts so we can then bring our attention back into the present. Through mindfulness practices, individuals are ultimately able to intentionally defuse from their thoughts, rather than allowing their thoughts to unknowingly dictate their emotional experience.

There are a variety of specific practices in any mindfulness intervention. This book covers those that are most relevant and accessible to the school-age population and that address all three axioms, as described previously. These include mindful breathing, meditation, gratitude practices, and yoga. Each of these is covered in detail in Chapter 3, along with hands-on practical techniques to use with youth at various developmental levels.

What Are Acceptance and Commitment Practices?

Acceptance involves choosing to make contact with difficult experiences, rather than avoiding them, struggling with them, or remaining painfully stuck. Whereas more traditional cognitive-behavioral modalities suggest that change occurs through such techniques as thought replacement or reinterpreting the meaning of a situation, acceptance practices approach situations with an open, flexible, and nonjudgmental posture combined with mindful awareness (Hayes et al., 2012). Once we accept our current situation or circumstance, we can then take committed action to make change via goals that are in keeping with our values. This approach has been coined acceptance and commitment therapy, or ACT. This theory is explored in greater detail in Chapter 4.

Why Use Mindfulness and ACT Practices in the Schools?

Between 2006–2016, there were over 350 randomized controlled research studies published on the positive effects of mindfulness (Creswell, 2017). Across most studies, participants were trained in present moment awareness but were not directly taught how to address negative thoughts (Creswell, 2017; Ludwig & Kabat-Zinn, 2008). However, as research has consistently shown that negative cognitive processes, such as rumination, are associated with increased internalizing (Peled & Moretti, 2010; Sibinga et al., 2013) and externalizing concerns Peled & Moretti, 2010), further attention has been focused on interventions that directly address an individual's relationship with their thoughts (e.g., acceptance-based strategies). The more recent integration of acceptance and mindfulness-based practices has been shown to be increasingly effective in combination, compared to when either strategy is used in isolation. For example, Chin et al. (2019) compared mindfulness training to mindfulness and acceptance training. Results indicated that the addition of acceptance-based strategies was a necessary active ingredient in improved treatment outcomes. Thus, incorporating both mindfulness and acceptance-based strategies into school-based interventions will likely optimize the benefits to students.

Although the literature has historically focused on use of mindfulness and ACT-based practices with adults, more recent research has examined its utility when working with youth in a variety of settings, including in the schools. Results of these studies have demonstrated that mindfulness and ACT practices are effective interventions for youth with a variety of presenting concerns, both physical and psychological (Ludwig & Kabat-Zinn, 2008). In fact, these practices are considered to be *transdiagnostic*, as they have broad applicability and demonstrated benefit across a variety of clinical presentations and levels of impairment (Swain et al., 2015). Specific to a school setting, numerous studies have now been published examining the effects of classroom-based mindfulness programs and have concluded that this approach results in improved mood and cognitive performance, as well as decreased stress and aggression (Creswell, 2017). Of importance, these strategies have been found to be equally effective among ethnic minority students and those from low socioeconomic backgrounds. For example, one large RCT examined the use of classroom-based mindfulness and acceptance-based interventions with a predominantly Black, low income, and urban middle school population. Results concluded that students experienced improved mood, increased effective coping, and decreased cognitive biases following participation in these interventions (Sibinga et al., 2016).

Just as importantly, these strategies have also been shown to promote the well-being of youth in the community at large (Creswell, 2017). In fact, the broad applicability of these practices is one of the primary advantages of using this approach in the school setting. According to Gillard et al. (2018), the benefits of using ACT and mindfulness-based interventions in the schools are threefold: for educators, the general population of students, and students with mental health concerns. Specific to educators, studies have found that when educators participate in learning these strategies, they report reduced stress and burnout, greater efficacy in their jobs, better classroom organization, and increased ability to promote a classroom environment that is emotionally supportive (Klingbeil & Renshaw, 2018). With regard to the general student population, research has concluded that schools using ACT and mindfulness-based strategies school-wide or in the classrooms results in students with improved focus and academic engagement, increased empathy and perspective taking, and enhanced resiliency (McKeering & Hwang, 2019; Napoli et al., 2005). Students with mental health concerns have also been shown to benefit from mindfulness and ACT-based interventions provided in a group or individual format (Chi et al., 2018; Livheim et al., 2014). Taken together, implementing school-based mindfulness and ACT-based programs can help promote the social and emotional well-being of all students and educators, while also working to change the developmental trajectory of those with mental health concerns through preventative and early intervention efforts.

A Look Ahead

This book follows an MTSS structure (see Figure 1.1), with chapters that respectively describe prevention and intervention efforts aimed at

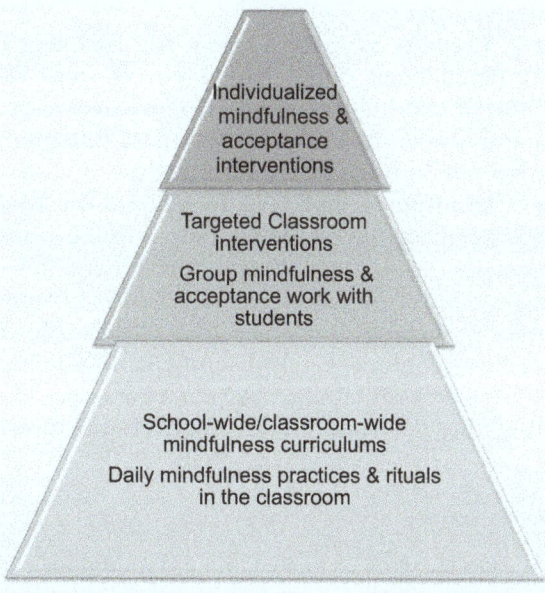

Figure 1.1 MTSS Model of Mindfulness and Acceptance-Based Practices in the School.

addressing the mental health concerns of youth in the schools at all three levels of support: schoolwide and class-wide, small group, and individualized treatments. Following is an overview of the remaining chapters.

- **Chapter 2: Research on Mindfulness and ACT Interventions.** This chapter reviews the research literature on the use of mindfulness and ACT practices with specific clinical populations and in the schools. It also discusses areas where additional research is needed.
- **Chapter 3: Mindfulness Techniques for Individual Work.** This chapter describes specific mindfulness techniques that can be used when providing individual intervention.
- **Chapter 4: ACT Strategies for Individual Work.** This chapter describes ACT techniques, particularly as they intersect with mindfulness strategies, that can be used when providing individual intervention.
- **Chapter 5: Mindfulness and ACT Strategies for Small Group Work.** This chapter introduces planning for and implementing group-based intervention. It details an eight-week mindfulness and ACT based group curriculum for use in the school setting.
- **Chapter 6: Mindfulness and ACT Strategies for Classroom and School-Wide Programming**. This chapter overviews mindfulness and

ACT practices that can be implemented in the classroom and/or as a school-wide program.

- **Chapter 7: Creating Systemic Change and Adapting Practices for Different Populations.** This chapter covers steps for increasing acceptability of mindfulness and ACT practices in the school setting and adapting these practices for a variety of different populations. Cultural considerations are also examined.
- **Chapter 8: Mindfulness and ACT Techniques for Adult Stakeholders.** This chapter focuses on the use of mindfulness and acceptance-based practices for teachers, parents, and other adult stakeholders, including specific resources for school-based intervention.
- **Chapter 9: Evaluating Outcomes and Conclusion**. This chapter describes how to monitor effectiveness of mindfulness and ACT practices in the school setting, provides an overview of material covered throughout this book, and highlights future directions.

References

Albrecht, N. J., Albrecht, P. M., & Cohen, M. (2012). Mindfully teaching in the classroom: A literature review. *Australian Journal of Teacher Education, 37*(12), 1–14.

California Department of Education. (2020, February 12). *Mental health services program overview: Mental health services in schools include a broad range of services, settings, and strategies.* www.cde.ca.gov/ls/cg/mh/mentalhealth.asp

Carballo, J. J., Baca-Garcia, E., Blanco, C., Perez-Rodriguez, M. M., Jimenez Arriero, M. A., Artes-Rodriguez, A., the members of Group for the Study of Evolution of Diagnosis (SED), Rynn, M., Shaffer, D., & Oquendo, M. A. (2010). Stability of childhood anxiety disorder diagnoses: A follow-up naturalistic study in psychiatric care. *European Child & Adolescent Psychiatry, 19*(4), 395–403.

Centers for Disease Control and Prevention. (2013). Mental health surveillance among children – United States, 2005–2011. *MMWR*, 1–35. www.cdc.gov/mmwr/preview/mmwrhtml/su6202a1.htm?s_cid=su6202a1_w

Chi, X., Bo, A., Liu, T., Zhang, P., & Chi, I. (2018). Effects of mindfulness-based stress reduction on depression in adolescents and young adults: A systematic review and meta-analysis. *Frontiers in Psychology, 9*, 1034.

Chin, B., Lindsay, E. K., Greco, C. M., Brown, K. W., Smyth, J. M., Wright, A. G. C., & Creswell, J. D. (2019). Psychological mechanisms driving stress resilience in mindfulness training: A randomized controlled trial. *Health Psychology, 38*(8), 759–768.

Creswell, J. D. (2017). Mindfulness Interventions. *Annual Review of Psychology, 68*, 491–516. https://doi.org/10.1146/annurev-psych-042716-051139

Daugherty, A. (2014). *From mindfulness to heartfulness: A journey of transformation through the science of embodiment.* Balboa Press.

Gillard, D., Flaxman, P., & Hooper, N. (2018). Acceptance and commitment therapy: Applications for educational psychologists within schools. *Educational Psychology in Practice, 34*(3), 272–281.

Hayes, S. C., Strosahl, K. D., & Wilson, K. G. (2012). *Acceptance and commitment therapy: An experiential approach to behavior change* (2nd ed.). Guilford Press.

Holland, M. L., Malmberg, J., & Gimpel Peacock, G. (2017). *Emotional and behavioral problems of young children: Effective interventions in the preschool and kindergarten year* (2nd ed.). Guilford Press.

Hong, J. S., Tillman, R., & Luby, J. L. (2015). Disruptive behavior in preschool children: Distinguishing normal misbehavior from markers of current and later childhood conduct disorder. *The Journal of Pediatrics, 166*(3), 723–730.

Kabat-Zinn, J. (1994). *Wherever you go, there you are: Mindfulness meditation in everyday life.* Hyperion.

Klingbeil, D. A., & Renshaw, T. L. (2018). Mindfulness-based interventions for teachers: A meta-analysis of the emerging evidence base. *School Psychology Quarterly, 33*(4), 501–511.

Livheim, F., Hayes, L., Ghaderi, A., Magnusdottir, T., Högfeldt, A., Rowse, J., Turner, S., Hayes, S. C., & Tengström, A. (2014). The effectiveness of acceptance and commitment therapy for adolescent mental health: Swedish and Australian pilot outcomes. *Journal of Child and Family Studies, 24*(4), 1016–1030.

Ludwig, D. S., & Kabat-Zinn, J. (2008). Mindfulness in medicine. *Journal of the American Medical Association, 300*(11), 1350–1352.

McKeering, P., & Hwang, Y. S. (2019). A systematic review of mindfulness-based school interventions with early adolescents. *Mindfulness, 10,* 593–610.

Mindful Schools. (2015a). *Mindfulness fundamentals.* www.mindfulschools.org/training/mindfulness-fundamentals/

Napoli, M., Krech, P. R., & Holley, L. C. (2005). Mindfulness training for elementary school students: The Attention Academy. *Journal of Applied School Psychology, 21*(1), 99–125.

National Association of School Psychologists. (2016). *School-based mental health services: Improving student learning and well-being.* www.nasponline.org/resources-and-publications/resources-and-podcasts/mental-health/school-psychology-and-mental-health/school-based-mental-health-services

National Institute of Medicine. (2009). *Preventing mental, emotional, and behavioral disorders among young people: Progress and possibilities.* Committee on Prevention of Mental Disorders and Substance Abuse Among Children, Youth, and Young Adults: Research Advances and Promising Interventions. The National Academies Press.

Peled, M., & Moretti, M. M. (2010). Ruminating on rumination: Are rumination on anger and sadness differentially related to aggression and depressed mood? *Journal of Psychopathology and Behavioral Assessment, 32*(1), 108–117.

Rechtschaffen, D. (2016). *The mindful education workbook: Lessons for teaching mindfulness to students.* W.W. Norton & Company.

Riddle, M. A., Yershova, K., Lazzaretto, D., Paykina, N., Yenokyan, G., Greenhill, L., Abikoff, H., Vitiello, B., Wigal, T., McCracken, J. T., Kollins, S. H., Murray, D. W., Wigal, S., Kastelic, E., McGough, J. J., dosReis, S., Bauzo-Rosario, A., Stehli, A., & Posner, K. (2013). The preschool attention-deficit/hyperactivity disorder treatment study (PATS) 6-year follow-up. *Journal of the American Academy of Child & Adolescent Psychiatry, 52*(3), 264–278.

Rones, M., & Hoagwood, K. (2000). School-based mental health services: A research review. *Clinical Child & Family Psychology Review, 3*(4), 223–241.

Salerno, J. P. (2016). Effectiveness of universal school-based mental health awareness programs among youth in the United States: A systematic review. *The Journal of school health, 86*(12), 922–931.

Sanchez, A. L., Cornacchio, D., Poznanski, B., Golik, A. M., Chou, T., & Comer, J. S. (2018). The effectiveness of school-based mental health services for elementary-aged children: A meta-analysis. *Journal of the American Academy of Child & Adolescent Psychiatry, 57*(3), 153–165.

Shapiro, S. L., Carlson, L. E., Astin, J. A., & Freedman, B. (2006). Mechanisms of mindfulness. *Journal of Clinical Psychology, 62*(3), 373–386.

Sibinga, E. M., Perry-Parrish, C., Chung, S. E., Johnson, S. B., Smith, M., & Ellen, J. M. (2013). School-based mindfulness instruction for urban male youth: A small randomized controlled trial. *Preventive Medicine, 57*(6), 799–801.

Sibinga, E. M., Webb, L., Ghazarian, S. R., & Ellen J. M. (2016). School-based mindfulness instruction: An RCT. *Pediatrics, 137*(1), 2015–2532.

Slemming, K., Sørensen, M. J., Thomsen, P. H., Obel, C., Henriksen, T. B., & Linnet, K. M. (2010). The association between preschool behavioural problems and internalizing difficulties at age 10–12 years. *European Child & Adolescent Psychiatry, 19*(10), 787–795.

Swain, J., Hancock, K., Dixon, A., & Bowman, J. (2015). Acceptance and commitment therapy for children: A systematic review of intervention studies. *Journal of Contextual Behavioral Science, 4*(2), 73–85.

Tolle, E. (1999). *The power of now: A guide to spiritual enlightenment.* New World Library.

U.S. Public Health Service. (2000). *Report of the surgeon general's conference on children's mental health: A national action agenda.* Department of Health and Human Services.

Werner-Seidler, A., Perry, Y., Calear, A. L., Newby, J. M., & Christensen, H. (2017). School-based depression and anxiety prevention programs for young people: A systematic review and meta-analysis. *Clinical Psychology Review, 51*, 30–47.

2 Research on Mindfulness and ACT Interventions

Roadmap to Chapter 2:

This chapter reviews the empirical literature on both mindfulness and ACT interventions. Specifically, the chapter covers:

- An overview of mindfulness research
- An overview of ACT research
- Mindfulness and use of technology
- Mindfulness and ACT with parents and teachers
- Challenges in empirical support for mindfulness practices

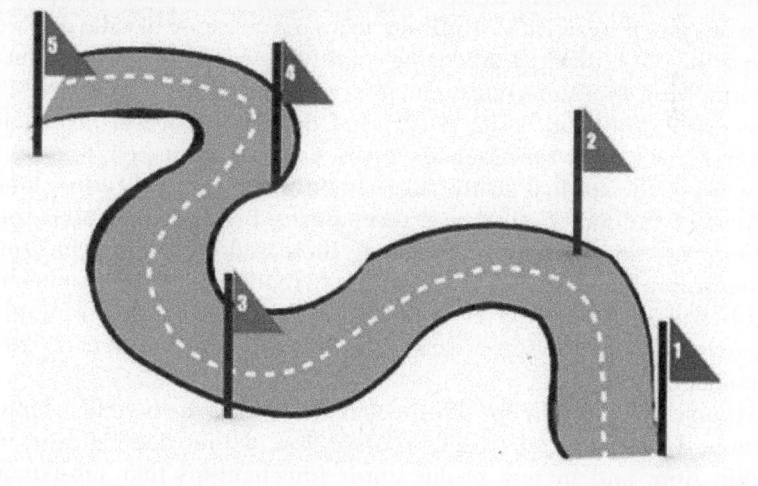

The first part of this chapter will overview mindfulness and acceptance-based practices and the research supporting their use. Specific areas of research include mindfulness with trauma-exposed youth, those with ADHD, at-risk youth, and young children (ages 4–6). The latter half

DOI: 10.4324/9781003318101-2

of the chapter examines research on mindfulness and ACT with adult stakeholders and the limitations of the current research.

Overview of Mindfulness Research

Mindfulness, or attending to the present moment without judgment, has been used as a secular Western therapeutic intervention over the last several decades. In general, research on mindfulness has shown positive benefits, including reduced stress and anxiety, improved immune functioning, improved emotional regulation, and overall improved mental health (Hanson & Mendius, 2009; National Center for Complementary and Integrative Medicine, 2017). These benefits are physical and mental, as well as structural. For example, the practice of mindfulness in adults has been found to alter the organization and action of neural circuitry in the brain that is associated with changes in stress reactivity and immune functioning (Davidson et al., 2003). Structural changes in the brain have been found in the prefrontal and parietal cortices (necessary for planning, decision making and impulse control) and the hippocampus (critical to learning and memory; Lazar et al., 2000). Research has supported the use of mindfulness-based interventions in helping to decrease resting blood pressure rates and to benefit the cardiovascular functioning of those at risk for hypertension (Barnes et al., 2001; Gregoski et al., 2011). These changes in brain functioning, along with decreased sympathetic nervous system reactivity, contribute to an overall sense of calm and well-being for the individual practicing mindfulness. This includes reduced internalizing symptoms such as anxiety and depression (Hanson & Mendius, 2009; Vøllestad et al., 2012), and decreased cortisol production (Brand et al., 2012; Sanada et al., 2016). Cortisol is released in response to stress by the adrenal glands (the structure that produces adrenaline), as part of the fight-flight-freeze mechanism. It causes increased respiration rates and increased heart rate. Increased cortisol production is strongly implicated in anxiety disorders (Sanada et al., 2016) and acting out behaviors (Schechter et al., 2012). Mindfulness has been found to decrease cortisol levels in otherwise healthy subjects (Brand et al., 2012; Sanada et al., 2016).

When examining the specific mechanism behind the benefits of mindfulness, Querstret and Cropley (2013) found that decreasing worry, rumination, and mental proliferation (mechanisms that substantially contribute to mental illness) significantly helped to reduce internalizing symptoms. Rumination has been linked to anxiety, with mindfulness practices linked to a reduction in ruminative thoughts and related anxiety (Sibinga et al., 2013). Mindfulness practices, specifically the focus on the present moment, have been found to interrupt maladaptive thinking patterns and contribute to the healing process by reducing negative types of thinking (Querstret & Cropley, 2013). In a meta-analysis conducted by Chi et al. (2018), 18 randomized controlled studies featuring over 2,000 teen and young adult participants found mindfulness interventions, relative to controls (e.g., no treatment, treatment as usual, or active control), had moderate effects in reducing depressive symptoms at the end of the intervention, though no significant effects were found at follow-up. In general, the longer the treatment intervention, the more significant the effects on participants' depressive symptoms. Therefore, it could be argued that longer treatments or booster sessions may be useful in maintaining gains.

To date, there are more studies examining mindfulness intervention with adults than with youth. Meta-analyses examining the effects of mindfulness with adults have evidenced therapeutic benefit for a variety of psychological problems, ranging from small to large effects. Table 2.1 contains a summary of these findings. Note for these studies, effect sizes are used which tells us how much one group differs from another – usually a difference between an experimental group and control group ranging from no effect, small effect, medium effect, and large effect. A meta-analysis is a statistical analysis that combines the results of multiple scientific studies.

Table 2.1 Key findings from meta-analyses on mindfulness with adults.

Author	Description	Sample	Effect Size
Khoury et al. (2013)	A meta-analysis of 209 published and unpublished studies examining the effects of mindfulness in participants with physical/medical conditions, psychological disorders, and non-clinical participants.	$N = 12,145$	waitlist-controlled studies: medium effect pre-post studies: medium effect active treatment studies: small to medium effect
Khoury et al. (2015)	A meta-analysis of 29 studies examining the effects of mindfulness in non-clinical participants.	$N = 2,668$	stress reduction: large effect depression, anxiety, distress reduction, and quality of life indicators: medium effect
Chen et al. (2012)	A meta-analysis of 40 randomized-controlled studies examining the effects of mindfulness on anxiety.	$N = 2,466$	burnout: small effect waitlist controlled studies: medium effect

Mindfulness With Youth

Research suggests that mindfulness practices can be effectively adapted for youth (Zelazo & Lyons, 2012). A recent meta-analysis conducted by Dunning et al. (2019) found mindfulness-based interventions, including meditation, mindful breathing, gratitude practices, and mindful movement, to be beneficial across all randomized controlled trials with youth. There were small to medium effect sizes in a variety of areas including: executive functioning, attention, depression, anxiety/stress, and disruptive behaviors. For those studies that included an active control group, improvements were seen particularly in the areas of depression, anxiety, and stress, with medium effect sizes found. These results are encouraging for the use of mindfulness as an intervention, particularly for internalizing disorders.

A number of studies have focused on the effects of specific mindfulness practices with youth. In particular, mindful breathing, meditation, yoga, and mindful movement have been a primary focus in studies of mindfulness with youth. The research behind these practices will be overviewed next.

Breathwork is considered the cornerstone of most mindfulness practices. Mindful breathing on its own has been shown to improve attention and reduce anxiety in youth. In a study by Telles et al. (2019), pre-adolescent children who engaged in yogic breathing significantly improved attention and reduced anxiety. In another study, 60 adolescents used pranaymama breathing (a form of yogic mindful breath) for 45 minutes, whereas the control group engaged in normal breathing. The heart rates and blood pressures, along with other physiological measures, were significantly reduced in those in the experimental group engaged in the breathwork, as compared to the controls (Kuppusamy et al., 2016).

Meditation practices are a more formal type of mindfulness. When practiced by children between the ages of 9–17 with internalizing symptoms, meditation has been found to help decrease anxiety and depression and to help improve attention and academic performance (Beauchemin et al., 2008; Semple et al., 2010; Raes et al., 2014). A study conducted by Schonert-Reichl and Lawlor (2010) found that a mindfulness meditation program for fourth through seventh graders resulted in improved self-reported optimism, positive affect, student attention, social-emotional competence, and externalizing behavior. Liehr and Diaz (2010), studied 8- to 11-year-old children in the Mindful Schools program (Mindful Schools, 2015a), which consisted of a combination of meditation and mindful breathing practices. Children in the mindfulness program had significantly lower levels of self-reported depressive symptoms on the Short Mood and Feelings Questionnaire (SMFQ; Angold et al., 1995) compared to those students in the health education only group (Liehr & Diaz, 2010).

Yoga has also been found to reduce anxiety in elementary aged children (Stueck & Gloeckner, 2005), with one study finding decreased cortisol levels and improved behaviors in second graders after participating in a 10-week yoga intervention (Butzer et al., 2015). Bazzano and colleagues (2018) found that third grade students who practiced yoga in the classroom significantly improved in anxiety and stress management compared to the control group. Yoga has also been implicated in helping children with pain management and major medical conditions (Moody et al., 2017), along with reducing the anxiety and depression associated with disordered eating in adolescents (Carei et al., 2010). In another study in a rural high school, students randomized to a semester of yoga (as opposed to their regular physical education (PE) curriculum) were found to either maintain or improve their stress levels, anxiety, anger control and negative affect, and resiliency, whereas those in the regular PE condition deteriorated in the area of negative affect (Noggle et al., 2012). In examining other forms of mindful movement, Wall (2005) found a five-week tai chi and mindfulness-based stress reduction program in a Boston public middle school helped to foster a sense of self-reported calmness, relaxation, improved sleep, less reactivity, increased self-care and self-awareness, and overall well-being in students.

In sum, mindfulness practices, including breathwork, meditation, and yoga, have been found to improve the mental and physical well-being of youth. Harnett and Dawe (2012) in their review of several dozen studies concluded that mindfulness-based interventions are an important addition to the repertoire of existing therapies when working with youth, particularly if parents can also participate to support these practices (Chapter 8 will cover mindfulness and acceptance practices with parents).

Mindfulness Research on Specific Youth Populations

Mindfulness has been found to be helpful for specific youth subgroups. In this section, we will review the recent research for four groups: youth who have experienced trauma, youth with attention problems, youth at risk of harming themselves or others, and young children (ages 4–6). Research related to the effects of mindfulness on academic performance will also be explored. The majority of the following studies were based on interventions with youth in the schools.

Trauma and Stress-Related Disorders

There is evidence that mindfulness-based practices may be effective in treating Post-Traumatic Stress Disorder (PTSD) in school-aged children (Catani et al., 2009). Mendelson et al. (2010) studied 97 fourth and fifth graders in a 12-week mindfulness program. Students were predominantly from low-income neighborhoods with high levels of violence and chronic stressors. Results indicated significant improvement for children in the program with regard to rumination, intrusive thoughts, and emotional arousal compared to the control group. Iacona and Johnson (2018) researched the neurobiological effects of mindfulness interventions on those who had experienced trauma, such as personal violence, natural disasters, and accidents. The researchers concluded that mindfulness interventions positively influenced children's ability to self-regulate and build resiliency. In a meta-analysis of 11 mindfulness studies containing comparable interventions and control groups, Kallapiran and colleagues (2015) found mindfulness-based interventions to be effective in improving anxiety and stress in comparison to non-active control groups.

Breath is also affected by trauma and the fear response. Zelano et al. (2016), studied the respiration, nervous system activation, and brain processes of 60 participants. Findings revealed that participants who engaged in rapid breathing, particularly through the nose with increased inhalation versus exhalation, demonstrated greater recognition of fearful stimuli and heightened arousal and vigilance. This process can be useful when someone is in a dangerous situation, leading to hypervigilance and nervous system activation (flight/fight/freeze phenomenon). However, for an individual with PTSD symptoms, this persistently activated state can become maladaptive and detrimental. In research examining nervous system activation, breathing exercises have been found to normalize parasympathetic activity in persons with anxiety (Asmundson & Stein, 1994). A research study by Walker and Pacik (2017) found that controlled, yogic breathing can help to reduce symptoms of PTSD.

Foster youth and those living in urban settings have been found to have increased trauma exposure, and therefore a higher incidence of stress, anxiety, and PTSD-related symptoms over the general childhood population (Breslau et al., 2004). Sibinga et al. (2013) studied a mindfulness-based stress reduction (MBSR) program in seventh and eighth grade urban males. Compared to the control group, participants in the MBSR program had less rumination, less anxiety, and fewer negative coping strategies after participating in the intervention. Cortisol levels, a common indicator of physiological stress, remained constant during the academic semester for the MBSR participants, whereas they increased for those in the control group. Jee et al. (2015) conducted a pilot study examining an MBSR program among 42 traumatized youth in foster and kinship care over 10 weeks. Youth, via self-report, indicated more competence in using their new strategies to manage ongoing stress and enhanced self-awareness post-intervention. In a related study by Sibinga et al. (2016), 300 low-income, minority, public middle school students were provided with either MBSR or a health education program. Students who participated in the MBSR program had significantly lower levels of depression and negative affect, rumination, somatization, negative coping, self-hostility, and posttraumatic symptom severity than those students in the health program. Though mindfulness-based practices may not replace more conventional approaches to treating trauma-related symptoms, such as trauma-focused CBT, these studies are promising and warrant ongoing investigation into the added utility of these interventions with this population (NCCIH, 2017).

Attention-Deficit/Hyperactivity Disorder (ADHD)

Mindfulness practices and yoga are now being incorporated into the repertoire of treatments for children and adolescents with ADHD. Klatt et al. (2012), studied mindfulness techniques, including meditation and breathwork, incorporated into a third-grade classroom at a low-income elementary school. After the intervention, the teachers reported fewer inattentive and hyperactive behaviors from the children. Similarly with adolescents, mindfulness training was found to increase attention and mindful awareness, while decreasing behavioral problems commonly associated with ADHD (van de Weijer-Bergsma et al., 2012). Jha and colleagues (2007) found that on performance tasks, mindfulness training enhances the functioning of participants to orient attention and improve attention-related behavioral responses.

Yoga has also been found helpful as an intervention for children with ADHD symptoms. In a study examining the use of a six-week yoga intervention with both parents and their children, those children with ADHD had a reduction in symptoms and improved self-esteem and relational functioning. Parents also reported feeling less stressed and better able to manage their child's behavior (Harrison et al., 2004). Jensen and Kenny (2004) studied yoga used as a complementary treatment in combination with medication for children with ADHD and found that yoga improved both attention and behavior. In a meta-analysis of studies including 5- to17-year-olds with ADHD, Chimiklis et al. (2018) found meditation, mindfulness-based practices, and/or yoga demonstrated statistically significant outcomes on improvement of ADHD symptoms, as well as executive functioning and parent-child relationships. However, given the risk for bias in these studies, they cautioned mindfulness-based therapies should not be considered a first-line intervention until more research validates its efficacy.

Youth At Risk for Harm

Mindfulness has also been found helpful with youth who are at risk of being a danger to themselves or others. Mindfulness practices can reduce some of the symptoms and risk factors associated with harm risk behaviors, such as reducing depressive symptoms (Liehr & Diaz, 2010;

Raes et al., 2014), increasing emotional regulation (Metz et al., 2013), and decreasing stress (Barnes et al., 2001). For those youth who have suicidal ideation or engage in non-suicidal self-injurious (NSSI) behaviors, Hayes and colleagues (2006) note that by increasing the youth's mindfulness of their psychological processes, they can reduce their desire to engage in experiential avoidance of psychological pain, a key function of both NSSI and suicidal behaviors. Therefore, the youth is equipped with a means of coping with the pain via mindfulness instead of engaging in self-harm behaviors. Additionally, stress-reduction, self-compassion, and living in the present moment can all be fostered when using mindfulness (Luoma & Villatte, 2012), thereby acting as protective factors against self-harm.

For youth who are at risk for harm to others, mindfulness has been shown to increase empathy and perspective taking (Schonert-Reichl et al., 2015) and have a calming effect in stressful situations (Chiesa & Serretti, 2009), all of which have been found to be protective factors when gauging violence risk. Mindfulness has also been found to decrease reactivity toward others (Goldin & Gross, 2010). A review of the related literature showed that mindfulness is particularly appropriate for intervening with anger due to its interrupting of negative cognitions, reducing physiological reactivity, and engendering positive mood (Wright et al., 2009).

Young Children

Research on the use of mindfulness with young children has also shown promising results. A study using a 12-week mindfulness-based kindness curriculum with preschool children showed students in the intervention group had greater improvements in social competence and earned higher report card grades in domains of health, learning, and social-emotional development than the control group at post-intervention (Flook et al., 2013). In another study, the effects of a 6-week mindfulness-based program (Head-Toes-Knees-Shoulders; HTKS) of 127 children (ages 4 to 6) in 8 kindergarten classrooms were compared to a control group. The teacher version of the Strengths and Difficulties Questionnaire (SDQ) was used to assess prosocial behavior and hyperactivity. Pre-post results indicated that children in the HTKS group were more prosocial, showed greater improvement in self-regulation, and were rated as having fewer hyperactive behaviors via teacher rating on the SDQ compared to children in the control group after the intervention (Viglas & Perlman, 2018). In addition to mindfulness, yoga has also been found to enhance young children's self-regulation. In a study by Razza and colleagues (2015), a year-long mindfulness yoga intervention implemented by the classroom teacher evidenced significant effect on preschool children's self-regulation, with those students at risk for problems in self-regulation benefiting the most. These findings provide promising support for the use of mindfulness and yoga in promoting prosocial behavior and self-regulation in young children in the schools.

Academic Performance and Mindfulness

Some research has also supported mindfulness practices in boosting academic functioning and performance in the classroom. This boost from mindfulness may be related to both the mindful student's ability to attend to a task without shifting attention (sustained attention) and also via the reduction of state anxiety, which has been implicated in poorer academic outcomes (Roodenrys et al., 2017).

Various studies have demonstrated the positive impact that mindfulness has on a child's executive functioning abilities (e.g., planning, attention, working memory, self-monitoring, and self-regulation, including inhibiting impulsivity). Numerous studies have also found improved attention for individuals who practice mindfulness, including better performance on tasks that require sustained attention (Chiesa & Serretti 2009; Jha, et al., 2007; Sedlmeier et al., 2012). See Table 2.2 for a summary of key findings in these areas.

Given the positive relationship between mindfulness, executive functioning, and attentional control, researchers have also postulated that students who practice mindfulness may also demonstrate improved academic achievement. Several studies summarized in Table 2.2 support this idea with students with learning disabilities, general education students, and undergraduate students. Mindfulness research has also been conducted with marginalized adolescents who are transitioning out of high school. Eva and Thayer (2017) studied 23 adolescents (ages 17 to 20, mostly males of color), using a six-week mindfulness-based intervention (Learning to Breathe curriculum; Broderick, 2013). Pre-post intervention survey responses revealed statistically significant differences in self-esteem and perceived stress, with the body scan technique being rated as the most optimal intervention. Improvement in the areas of self-regulation, attention-awareness, and positive thinking were noted by the participants. Other studies have confirmed these findings using this curriculum (Bluth et al., 2015). Taken together, mindfulness-based strategies appear to have utility when working with students across their academic careers.

Research on Mindfulness and Use of Technology

More recently, telehealth practices have been utilized in the school setting by school-related mental health professionals to deliver services to youth. The use of technology, such as video conferencing, online programs, and mobile phone applications, can be cost effective and increase

Table 2.2 Studies examining the association between executive functioning, attention, or academic performance and mindfulness.

Outcome Variable	Study	Sample Characteristics	Results
Executive Functioning	Flook et al. (2010)	$N = 64$ Grades = 2–3 Typically developing students in the U.S.	After receiving eight weeks of the Mindful Awareness Practices program participants, and especially those with low executive functioning, showed marked improvement in behavioral regulation, metacognition, and overall executive functioning.
	Lu et al. (2017)	$N = 219$ Grades = 5–7 Typically developing migrant students in China	Self-reported mindfulness was positively associated with executive functioning and academic performance.
	Oberle et al. (2012)	$N = 99$ Grades = 4–5 Typically developing students in Canada	Self-reported mindfulness was found to positively predict inhibitory control, controlling for grade, gender, and salivary morning cortisol levels.
Attention	Black and Fernando (2014)	$N = 409$ Grades = K – 6 Typically developing primarily low-income ethnic minority students in the U.S.	After receiving five weeks of a mindfulness-based curriculum, students showed greater attention, self-regulation, and active participation in class.
	Napoli et al. (2005)	$N = 194$ Grades = 1–3 Typically developing students in the U.S.	After receiving 24 weeks of a mindfulness-based curriculum, participants showed marked improvement on three measures of attention, compared to controls.
	Zenner et al. (2014)	$N = 1,348$ Grades = 1–12 Samples drawn from North America, Europe, Asia, and Australia	A meta-analysis of 24 studies revealed that mindfulness-based interventions showed large effect sizes in areas underlying cognitive performance, including attention.
Academic Performance	Beauchemin et al. (2008)	$N = 34$ Grades = 9–12 Students with learning disabilities from a private residential school in the U.S.	After a five-week mindfulness-based intervention, participants showed decreased state and trait anxiety, improved social skills, and academic performance.
	Mrazek et al. (2013)	$N = 48$ Grades = undergraduate Typically developing college students in the U.S.	After a two-week mindfulness-based intervention, participants showed higher GRE accuracy (16 points) and improved working memory capacity compared to those who received instruction in nutrition.

service accessibility to children and families that otherwise may not be able to participate (MacDonell & Prinz, 2017). Online mindfulness-based programs have been shown to significantly reduce stress and increase emotional regulation abilities in youth (Ma et al., 2018). In these programs, self-directed interventions, paired with online group discussions that offer the addition of social support, lead to improved mood and decreased stress. Though studies examining the effectiveness of these online approaches are still emerging, the few that have been conducted found overall positive results (Cavanagh et al., 2013; Ma et al., 2018).

In addition to online programs, the use of mobile phone applications (e.g., Headspace, Calm) have been shown to be effective supplements to intervention (Lucas-Thompson et al., 2019). Youth can access these applications on their phones whenever needed, day or night, to help support their well-being. Along these lines, mindfulness practice has also been combined with the delivery of structured or unstructured intervention through text messages (ecological momentary intervention; EMI; ecological momentary assessment; EMA). School-based professionals can create scheduled times for delivering the texted intervention, while also helping youth apply their learned skills within the context of the home environment. Lucas-Thompson et al. (2019) found improvement in the well-being of youth at risk for NSSI and suicidal ideation using mindfulness and EMI's. In a systematic review of current published research in this area, Malakouti and colleagues (2020) found that the use of mobile applications had an overall positive effect on reducing suicide risk and improving the health of participants. Though research in this area is still emerging, the use of phone apps appears to be promising for supporting school-based mental health intervention.

Overview of ACT Research

ACT is a form of cognitive-behavioral therapy that combines mindfulness with self-acceptance (O'Brien et al., 2008). As described in Chapter 1, the emphasis on acceptance of one's experiences through use of mindfulness and behavior change strategies increases the individual's psychological flexibility (Hayes et al., 2012). Once we accept our current circumstance, we can act to make change (Hayes et al., 2006).

ACT has been well documented over the last several decades for its use with adult populations. More recently, ACT has been adapted for use with youth. Given the relative recency of using ACT with youth, there are few studies to date examining its use in schools. However, given its applicability and effectiveness with youth in clinical and home settings, similar outcomes should be expected in the school setting. Table 2.3 summarizes a sampling of studies on ACT for youth mental health concerns.

When looking specifically at the school environment, ACT has been studied in the areas of stress and well-being. Stress and anxiety are

Table 2.3 Studies supporting treatment of childhood conditions with ACT.

Condition Targeted	Study	Sample	Results
Anxiety	Hancock et al. (2016)	$N = 111$	After a 10-week intervention, both groups assigned to the ACT and CBT intervention showed significant reduction in anxiety, with a non-significantly different 45% and 60% of ACT and CBT participants respectively remaining symptom free at two-year follow-up.
Eating Disorders	Heffner et al. (2002)	$N = 1$	A 15-year-old girl diagnosed with anorexia nervosa showed greater acceptance of weight-related cognitions and redirection of her desire for thinness into healthier goals following treatment with ACT combined with CBT.
Chronic Pain	Wicksell et al. (2007)	$N = 14$	14 adolescents with chronic pain were successfully treated using ACT, showing a 68% reduction in school days missed due to pain, a 63% decrease in functional disability, and increased psychological flexibility. 46% of participants also reported a significant reduction in pain. These gains were maintained at three- and six-month follow-up.
	Wicksell et al. (2011)	$N = 32$	After 10 weeks of individual ACT with parent support sessions, participants showed a significant reduction in pain-related disability, and life satisfaction which was mediated by psychological flexibility.
Repetitive and Restrictive Behaviors	Eilers and Hayes (2015)	Experiment 1: $N = 3$ Experiment 2: $N = 4$	Utilizing exposure therapy, combined with cognitive defusion techniques, participants diagnosed with autism showed a significant reduction in frequency of engaging in repetitive or restricted behavior.

common experiences for youth in the schools. Academic stress, including high stakes testing and large amounts of homework, has been identified as a common risk factor for students' increased anxiety levels (Galloway et al., 2013; Leung et al., 2010). Moreover, students who experience school-related stress tend to develop associated physical symptoms, such as headaches, fatigue, and sleeping difficulties (Galloway et al., 2013). Encouragingly, school-based ACT intervention has been found to significantly reduce student stress levels. In a study by Livheim et al. (2014), students rated themselves as having significantly less stress-related symptoms after an eight-session ACT group, as compared to a wait-list control group. Dixon (2013) reported positive initial outcomes resulting from a one-year ACT-based life-skills curriculum in a school setting, including increased attendance, improved well-being, and a reduction in reported behavioral concerns by teachers. The curriculum included universal components, which all students accessed, and more intensive and targeted components, accessed only by students experiencing specific emotional or behavioral challenges. Similarly, in a school-based study of ACT combined with Adventure Therapy (the use of outdoor adventures to increase team building and well-being) for children with behavioral and emotional problems, participants had increased self-calming, higher personal goal attainment, enhanced teamwork, and increased respect and trust for others (Tracey et al., 2018). Another research study on ACT examined 267 10th and 11th grade high-school students. Those in the ACT program, compared to controls, reported significant reductions in depression, stress, and composite depression/anxiety symptoms, with medium to strong effect sizes. This study suggests that including acceptance in early intervention programs may be effective in reducing symptoms and improving well-being in high school students (Burckhardt et al., 2016).

Mindfulness and ACT in Parent Work

Incorporating parents into their child's mental health treatment has many advantages, including increased treatment engagement, improved generalization of skills, and being able to address parenting factors that may be contributing to the child's presenting problems (Taylor & Adelman, 2001). Mindfulness and ACT techniques have been incorporated into parent work and parent training programs (Coyne & Murrell, 2009). Mindfulness-based strategies encourage parents to be present-focused and nonjudgmental toward their thoughts, feelings, and behaviors, as well as their child's behaviors. Studies have demonstrated that teaching mindfulness to parents improves parent psychopathology, reduces parenting stress, and results in increased use of effective parenting practices (Bögels & Restifo, 2014), all of which have been shown to influence child psychopathology. Table 2.4 summarizes examples of studies of mindfulness use with parents.

Table 2.4 Studies supporting the use of mindfulness with parents.

Child's Characteristics	Study	Sample	Results
Low-income	Mathis et al. (2018)	$N = 27$	After eight weeks of weekly mindful parenting sessions, parents reported decreased distress, sleep disturbances, and depressive symptoms, and increased parental support given to their children.
Developmental delays	Neece et al. (2013)	$N = 46$	Parents receiving a mindfulness-based stress reduction program reported fewer depressive symptoms and stress, greater life satisfaction, and fewer behavior problems in their child, especially in ADHD symptoms.
Autism	Singh et al. (2006)	$N = 3$	Mothers who were trained in a 12-week mindfulness program reported reductions in their child's levels of aggression, self-injury, and noncompliance, and increased satisfaction with their parenting skills and interactions with their children.
Chronic health conditions	Hou et al. (2014)	$N = 141$	Caregivers of family members with chronic health conditions who received an eight-week mindfulness-based stress reduction program reported reductions in state anxiety and reported self-efficacy in controlling negative thoughts and mindfulness. Reductions in anxiety did not persist at three-month follow-up.

Over the last decade more research has been conducted examining the use of ACT with parents. ACT interventions can support parents in increasing their psychological flexibility (e.g., reduced experiential avoidance and cognitive fusion), which in turn results in engagement in more effective parenting strategies. For example, parents can be taught to relate to their thoughts more effectively through use of cognitive defusion techniques, which in turn results in use of more effective parenting practices. Table 2.5 contains a sampling of examples of research on ACT and parenting.

The studies included in Table 2.5 provide initial empirical support for the use of ACT when working with parents. Following participation in ACT interventions, parents have reported improvement in their own mental health, improvement in the parent-child relationship, and engagement in more effective parenting strategies, all of which have

Table 2.5 Studies supporting the use of ACT with parents.

Child's Characteristics	Study	Sample	Results
Autism	Poddar et al. (2015)	$N = 5$	After 10 sessions of an ACT program, parents reported decreased state anxiety, depression, psychological flexibility, and better quality of life.
Cerebral palsy	Whittingham et al. (2016)	$N = 67$	After eight sessions of an ACT-based parent training program, parents reported increased child functional performance, quality of life, and decreased parental psychological symptoms.
Cancer/ Cardiac problems	Burke et al. (2014)	$N = 11$	Parents receiving an ACT-based intervention reported reductions in posttraumatic stress and emotional impact from their child's illness, and improvements in mindfulness and psychological flexibility. These effects were maintained at six-month follow-up.
Conduct problems	Coyne and Wilson (2004)	$N = 1$	After receiving treatment combining ACT and parent-child interaction therapy (PCIT), a mother of a six-year-old with conduct problems reported increased feelings of competence and parenting skills, lower child aggression and non-compliance, decreased parental anxiety, and increased self-efficacy in engaging in social interactions.

been shown to contribute to a reduction in childhood behavioral and emotional concerns (Coyne & Wilson, 2004; Holland et al., 2017).

Taken together, there is emerging literature supporting the use of ACT and mindfulness practices when working with parents. Through use of these interventions, parents can be supported in using mindfulness and behavior change strategies that result in improved psychological flexibility (i.e., having contact with the present moment and engaging in purposeful behaviors aligned with their parenting values; Hayes et al., 2012). In turn, parents experience improved psychological well-being, and engage in more effective parenting practices, all of which result in improved child behavioral and emotional well-being.

Mindfulness and ACT With Teachers

Mindfulness and ACT have more recently been researched with teachers, including in the areas of classroom management, teaching performance, and burnout prevention. It has been found that 46% of all new teachers in the United States leave the profession within five years, with the teacher drop-out rate higher than the student drop-out rate (Black et al., 2008). For example, in the 2012–2013 school year, 8% of teachers left the field (National Center for Education Statistics [NCES], 2015), with urban schools often experiencing even higher teacher turnover, up to 20% (National Commission on Teaching and America's Future [NCTAF], 2007). Research has shown teachers with higher stress levels have lower job satisfaction, which is also indirectly linked to their feelings of self-efficacy in classroom management and teaching performance (Klassen & Chiu, 2010). Therefore, interventions that help support teachers and prevent related burnout are crucial to creating stable and healthy classroom environments.

Mindfulness has been found to have positive results in aiding teachers in their classroom management and teaching performance. Table 2.6 summarizes per grade level some of the research examining the classroom-based effects of mindfulness use with teachers.

Given these findings summarized in Table 2.6, mindfulness can be considered a feasible, cost-effective method for reducing stress and improving performance for teachers.

Mindfulness and ACT not only help teachers in the classroom, but these strategies can also assist in their personal well-being. Table 2.7 contains a summary of the research on the impact of mindfulness and ACT on teacher well-being.

Teacher burnout is another area wherein mindfulness and ACT have been utilized. Table 2.8 contains a summary of the treatment effects

Table 2.6 Classroom-based effects of mindfulness with teachers.

Grade Level Taught	Study	Sample	Results
Preschool	Singh et al. (2013)	$N = 21$ $n = 3$ (teachers) $n = 18$ (students)	After receiving eight weeks of mindfulness-based training, teachers reported that their students showed fewer difficult behaviors and negative peer interactions, and increased compliance with directives.
Elementary	Flook et al. (2013)	$N = 18$	After participating in eight sessions of a mindfulness-based stress reduction program, teachers in the intervention group compared to control reported reductions in psychological distress, burnout, and improvements in observer-rated classroom organization and self-compassion.

Grade Level Taught	Study	Sample	Results
PreK– 12th grade	Taylor et al. (2016)	$N = 59$	After participating in a mindfulness-based training, teachers in the intervention group compared to control reported increased efficacy in regulating emotions and their tendency to forgive students. These factors partially mediated stress reduction at baseline and four-month follow-up.
	Jennings et al. (2013)	$N = 50$	After participating in a mindfulness-based training, teachers in the intervention group compared to control reported improvements in well-being, self-efficacy, burnout/ time-related stress, and mindfulness.

Table 2.7 Studies examining the impact of mindfulness and ACT on teacher well-being.

Intervention Type	Study	Sample	Results
Mindfulness	Emerson et al. (2017)	$N = 589$	Through a systematic review of 12 studies, it was found that mindfulness-based interventions with educators reduce stress primarily through improvements in decentering, regulation of attention, and self-compassion, which in turn enhances emotion regulation skills and teacher self-efficacy.
	Kerr et al. (2017)	$N = 23$	After engaging in a six-week mindfulness-based curriculum, preservice teachers in the intervention compared to the control group showed greater emotional clarity and regulation of negative emotions. Within-group differences suggest that mindfulness helped teachers control impulsive behaviors and respond more flexibly to stressful emotions.
ACT	Biglan et al. (2013)	$N = 42$	After engaging in a two session ACT-based workshop, early childhood special education teachers in the intervention compared to control group showed increased acceptance of inner experiences, reduced stress, and increased feelings of efficacy.

Table 2.8 Studies examining the effects of mindfulness and ACT on burnout.

Intervention Type	Study	Sample	Results
Mindfulness	Roeser et al. (2013)	N = 113	After engaging in an eight-week mindfulness training program, teachers in the intervention compared to the control group showed improved mindfulness, focused attention, working memory capacity, occupational self-compassion, and lower levels of occupational stress and burnout, with benefits persisting at three-month follow-up. Mediational analysis suggests that group differences in mindfulness and self-compassion mediated stress reduction, burnout, anxiety, and depression at follow-up.
	Sharp Donahoo et al. (2018)	N = 27	After engaging in a three-hour seminar on stress and compassion fatigue and the benefits of prayer, mindfulness, and social supports, participants who practiced mindfulness showed reduced perceived stress compared to educators who did not practice mindfulness.
	Flook et al. (2013)	N = 18	After participating in eight sessions of a mindfulness-based stress reduction program, teachers in the intervention group compared to control reported reductions in psychological distress, burnout, and improvements in observer-rated classroom organization and self-compassion.
ACT	Jeffcoat and Hayes (2012)	N = 236	After engaging in a 10-week ACT-based bibliotherapy program, educators in the intervention compared to the control group showed improved psychological health, including reduced stress, anxiety, and depressive symptoms, as well as improved mindfulness and psychological flexibility.
	Hinds et al. (2015)	N = 529	Found experiential avoidance is associated with burnout and depression.
	Lloyd et al. (2013)	N = 43	After intervention, psychological flexibility increased, and emotional exhaustion decreased compared to the control group.
	Brinkborg et al. (2011)	N = 106	After social workers engaged in ACT, participants experienced significantly decreased levels of stress and burnout, and increased general mental health.

on burnout in teachers. In general, mindfulness has shown promise for reducing burnout, with research supporting its use with teachers (Seney & Mishou, 2018).

Taken together, there is a strong emerging literature supporting the benefits of mindfulness and acceptance-based interventions on the well-being of youth, parents, and educators. Youth who participate in these interventions have been shown to demonstrate reduced emotional and behavioral difficulties, as well as improved academic performance. Following participation in these interventions, parents report improved parenting efficacy, reduced psychological distress, and enhanced quality of life. Educators experience benefits both with regard to their teaching performance, as well as to their personal psychological well-being, following use of mindfulness and ACT-based strategies. While these preliminary studies are promising, future research is needed, as further described next.

Challenges in Mindfulness Research

Mindfulness is considered a relatively new clinical intervention, and, though its roots are centuries old, only in the past several decades has it been used more widely as a psychotherapeutic intervention. Consequently, the research in this area is still developing. There are several current challenges in the literature regarding empirically evaluating the clinical utility of mindfulness. For example, there is no common consensus regarding the definition of mindfulness, making it difficult to operationalize, measure, and compare across studies (Eklund et al., 2017). Additional measurement difficulties have been encountered due to the internal nature of mindfulness processes (compared to observable behaviors). Thus, researchers must largely rely on self-report measures, which has inherent limitations, particularly when working with a younger population. Furthermore, few well-validated self-report mindfulness measures are available when working with youth. Concerns have also been raised that mindfulness questionnaires do not always correlate with the intervention used (Manuel et al., 2017), and the underlying latent variable influencing the item responses on certain scales may be reflective of some variable other than mindfulness, such as inattentiveness (Van Dam et al., 2010). Therefore, even those studies that inquire about levels of mindful awareness may be erroneously measuring the wrong variable. In addition to the challenges in measuring mindfulness via rating scales, neuroscience researchers must grapple with the limitations of neuroimaging methods (Van Dam et al., 2018).

In a meta-analytic review of the literature examining mindfulness studies with children, Zoogman and colleagues (2015) concluded that there are positive effects across studies, though the quality of the studies may undermine the confidence by which conclusions can be drawn

(Roodenrys et al., 2017). For example, many studies lack control groups (Schonert-Reichl et al., 2015; Van Dam et al., 2018). An additional challenge in researching mindfulness-based interventions is the common practice of incorporating other cognitive behavioral techniques into the comprehensive treatment protocol. As a result, it can be difficult to identify which treatment component directly impacted the treatment outcomes (e.g., the cognitive, behavioral, and/or mindfulness components; Manuel et al., 2017). Thus, additional research focused specifically on mindfulness-based interventions is needed to determine the impact these strategies have on pertinent outcomes.

The fidelity of implementation (FOI) of the intervention is also an issue when understanding mindfulness research. A review of the literature indicated a relative dearth of rigorous FOI in research, with fewer than 10% of studies outlining the potential core program components or theory of intervention, and fewer than 20% assessing any aspect of FOI beyond the amount of intervention implemented (Gould et al., 2015). Therefore, it is important that researchers attend to the integrity of the intervention when reporting results.

Conclusion and Future Directions

In general, mindfulness and ACT interventions have been found to be efficacious when working with students, parents, and teachers in a variety of areas, including stress reduction, treating internalizing disorders, increasing focus and attention, and supporting overall well-being. Though research is, in general, supportive of the use of mindfulness in educational settings, challenges with existing research and determining the efficacy of mindfulness practices rests on multiple factors, including the problem of defining mindfulness across studies, the lack of control groups, and issues in the methodological study of mindfulness itself. Therefore, more research must be conducted to better understand the utility of mindfulness in academic settings, with greater rigor involved in the methodology and study of these practices. That said, mindfulness and ACT have been supported by the research literature as an important addition to mental health intervention in school-aged youth, educators, and parents.

References

Angold, A., Costello, E. J., Messer, S. C., Pickles, A., Winder, F., & Silver, D. (1995). The development of a short questionnaire for use in epidemiological studies of depression in children and adolescents. *International Journal of Methods in Psychiatric Research, 5*(4), 237–249.

Asmundson, G. J., & Stein, M. B. (1994). Vagal attenuation in panic disorder: An assessment of parasympathetic nervous system function and subjective reactivity to respiratory manipulations. *Psychosomatic Medicine, 56*(3), 187–193.

Barnes, V. A., Treiber, F., & Davis, H. (2001). Impact of transcendental meditation ® on cardiovascular function at rest and during acute stress in adolescents with high normal blood pressure. *Journal of Psychosomatic Research, 51*(4), 597–605.

Bazzano, A. N., Anderson, C. E., Hylton, C., & Gustat, J. (2018). Effect of mindfulness and yoga on quality of life for elementary school students and teachers: Results of a randomized controlled school-based study. *Psychology Research and Behavior Management, 11*, 81–89. https://doi.org/10.2147/PRBM.S157503

Beauchemin, J., Hutchins, T. L., & Patterson, F. (2008). Mindfulness meditation may lessen anxiety, promote social skills, and improve academic performance among adolescents with learning disabilities. *Complementary Health Practice Review, 13*(1), 34–45.

Biglan, A., Layton, G. L., Jones, L. B., Hankins, M., & Rusby, J. C. (2013). The value of workshops on psychological flexibility for early childhood special education staff. *Topics in Early Childhood Special Education, 32*(4), 196–210.

Black, D. S., & Fernando, R. (2014). Mindfulness training and classroom behavior among lower-income and ethnic minority elementary school children. *Journal of Child and Family Studies, 23*(7), 1242–1246.

Black, L., Neel, J., & Benson, G. (2008). *National Commission on Teaching and America's Future (NCTAF)/Georgia State University (GSU) induction project: Final report* (ED504316). ERIC. http//eric.ed.gov/PDFS/ED504316.pdf

Bluth, K., Roberson, P. N., & Gaylord, S. A. (2015). A pilot study of a mindfulness intervention for adolescents and the potential role of self-compassion in reducing stress. *Explore, 11*(4), 292–295.

Bögels, S., & Restifo, K. (2014). *Mindful parenting: A guide for mental health practitioners.* W. W. Norton & Co.

Brand, S., Holsboer-Trachsler, E., Naranjo, J. R., & Schmidt, S. (2012). Influence of mindfulness practice on cortisol and sleep in long-term and short-term meditators. *Neuropsychobiology, 65*, 109–118.

Breslau, N., Wilcox, H. C., Storr, C. L., Lucia, V. C., & Anthony, J. C. (2004). Trauma exposure and posttraumatic stress disorder: A study of youths in urban America. *Journal of Urban Health, 81*(4), 530–544.

Brinkborg, H., Michanek, J., Hesser, H., & Berglund, G. (2011). Acceptance and commitment therapy for the treatment of stress among social workers: A randomized controlled trial. *Behaviour Research and Therapy, 49*(6–7), 389–398.

Broderick, P. C. (2013). *Learning to Breathe: About L2B.* https://learning2brea the.org/

Burckhardt, R., Manicavasagar, V., Batterham, P. J., & Hadzi-Pavlovic, D. (2016). A randomized controlled trial of strong minds: A school-based mental health program combining acceptance and commitment therapy and positive psychology. *Journal of School Psychology, 57*, 41–52.

Burke, K., Muscara, F., McCarthy, M., Dimovski, A., Hearps, S., Anderson, V., & Walser, R. (2014). Adapting acceptance and commitment therapy for parents of children with life-threatening illness: Pilot study. *Families, Systems, & Health, 32*(1), 122–127.

Butzer, B., van Over, M., Noggle Taylor, J. J., & Khalsa, S. B. S. (2015). Yoga may mitigate decreases in high school grades. *Evidence-Based Complementary and Alternative Medicine, 2015*, Article 259814, 1–8.

Carei, T. R., Fyfe-Johnson, A. L., Breuner, C. C., & Brown, M. A. (2010). Randomized controlled clinical trial of yoga in the treatment of eating disorders. *Journal of Adolescent Health, 46*(4), 346–351.

Catani, C., Kohiladevy, M., Ruf, M., Schauer, E., Elbert, T., & Neuner, F. (2009). Treating children traumatized by war and Tsunami: A comparison between exposure therapy and meditation-relaxation in North-East Sri Lanka. *BMC Psychiatry, 9*(1), 1–22.

Cavanagh, K., Strauss, C., Cicconi, F., Griffiths, N., Wyper, A., & Jones, F. A. (2013). Randomised controlled trial of a brief online mindfulness-based intervention. *Behaviour Research and Therapy, 51*(9), 573–578.

Chen, K. W., Berger, C. C., Manheimer, E., Forde, D., Magidson, J., Dachman, L., & Lejuez, C. W. (2012). Meditative therapies for reducing anxiety: A systematic review and meta-analysis of randomized controlled trials. *Depression and Anxiety, 29*(7), 545–562.

Chi, X., Bo, A., Liu, T., Zhang, P., & Chi, I. (2018). Effects of mindfulness-based stress reduction on depression in adolescents and young adults: A systematic review and meta-analysis. *Frontiers in Psychology, 9*, 1034.

Chiesa, A. L., & Serretti, A. (2009). Mindfulness-based stress reduction for stress management in healthy people: A review and meta-analysis. *Journal of Alternative Complementary Medicine, 15*(5), 593–600.

Chimiklis, A. L., Dahl, V., Spears, A. P., Goss, K., Fogarty, K., & Chacko, A. (2018). Yoga, mindfulness, and meditation interventions for youth with ADHD: Systematic review and meta-analysis. *Journal of Child and Family Studies, 27*(10), 3155–3168.

Coyne, L. W., & Murrell, A. R. (2009). *The joy of parenting: An acceptance and commitment therapy guide to effective parenting in the early years.* New Harbinger Publications.

Coyne, L. W., & Wilson, K. G. (2004). The role of cognitive fusion in impaired parenting: An RFT analysis. *International Journal of Psychology and Psychological Therapy, 4*(3), 469–486.

Davidson, R. J., Kabat-Zinn, J., Schumacher, J., Rosenkranz, M., Muller, D., Santorelli, S. F., Urbanowski, F., Harrington, A., Bonus, K., & Sheridan, J. F. (2003). Alterations in brain and immune function produced by mindfulness meditation. *Psychosomatic Medicine, 65*(4), 564–570.

Dixon, M. (2013). Don't stop believing: Journeys school. *Behaviour Analysis in Practice, 6*, 23–24.

Dunning, D. L., Griffiths, K., Kuyken, W., Crane, C., Foulkes, L., Parker, J., & Dalgleish, T. (2019). Research review: The effects of mindfulness-based interventions on cognition and mental health in children and adolescents – A meta-analysis of randomized controlled trials. *Journal of Child Psychology and Psychiatry, 60*(3), 244–258.

Eilers, H. J., & Hayes, S. C. (2015). Exposure and response prevention therapy with cognitive defusion exercises to reduce repetitive and restrictive behaviors displayed by children with autism spectrum disorder. *Research in Autism Spectrum Disorders, 19*, 18–31.

Eklund, K., O'Malley, M., & Meyer, L. (2017). Gauging mindfulness in children and youth: School-based applications. *Psychology in the Schools, 54*(1), 101–114.

Emerson, L. M., Leyland, A., Hudson, K., Rowse, G., Hanley, P., & Hugh-Jones, S. (2017). Teaching mindfulness to teachers: A systematic review and narrative synthesis. *Mindfulness, 8*(5), 1136–1149.

Eva, A. L., & Thayer, N. M. (2017). Learning to BREATHE: A pilot study of a mindfulness-based intervention to support marginalized youth. *Journal of Evidence-Based Complementary & Alternative Medicine, 22*(4), 580–591.

Flook, L., Goldberg, S. B., Pinger, L., Bonus, K., & Davidson, R. J. (2013). Mindfulness for teachers: A pilot study to assess effects on stress, burnout and teaching efficacy. *Mind Brain Education, 7*(3), 186–195.

Flook, L., Smalley, S. L., Kitil, M. J., Galla, B. M., Kaiser-Greenland, S., Locke, J., Ishijima, E., & Kasari, C. (2010). Effects of mindful awareness practices on executive functions in elementary school children. *Journal of Applied School Psychology, 26*(1), 70–95.

Galloway, M., Conner, J., & Pope, D. (2013). Nonacademic effects of homework in privileged, high-performing high schools. *The Journal of Experimental Education, 81*(4), 490–510.

Goldin, P. R., & Gross, J. J. (2010). Effects of mindfulness-based stress reduction (MBSR) on emotion regulation in social anxiety disorder. *Emotion, 10*(1), 83–91.

Gould, L. F., Dariotis, J. K., Greenberg, M. T., & Mendelson, T. (2015). Assessing fidelity of implementation (FOI) for school-based mindfulness and yoga interventions: A systematic review. *Mindfulness, 7*(1), 5–33.

Gregoski, M. J., Barnes, V. A., Tingen, M. S., Harshfield, G. A., & Treiber, F. A. (2011). Breathing awareness meditation and LifeSkills training programs influence upon ambulatory blood pressure and sodium excretion among African American adolescents. *Journal of Adolescent Health, 48*(1), 59–64.

Hancock, K., Swain, J., Hainsworth, C., Koo, S., & Dixon, A. (2016). Long term follow up in children with anxiety disorders treated with acceptance and commitment therapy or cognitive behavioral therapy: Outcomes and predictors. *Journal of Child and Adolescent Behavior, 4*, 317–330.

Hanson, R., & Mendius, R. (2009). *Buddha's brain: The practical neuroscience of happiness, love, and wisdom.* New Harbinger Publication.

Harnett, P. H., & Dawe, S. (2012). The contribution of mindfulness-based therapies for children and families and proposed conceptual integration. *Child and Adolescent Mental Health, 17*(4), 195–208.

Harrison, L. J., Manocha, R., & Rubia, K. (2004). Sahaja yoga meditation as a family treatment programme for children with attention deficit-hyperactivity disorder. *Clinical Child Psychology and Psychiatry, 9*(4), 479–497.

Hayes, S. C., Luoma, J. B., Bond, F. W., Masuda, A., & Lillis, J. (2006). Acceptance and commitment therapy: Model, processes and outcomes. *Behaviour Research and Therapy, 44*(1), 1–25.

Hayes, S. C., Strosahl, K. D., & Wilson, K. G. (2012). *Acceptance and commitment therapy: An experiential approach to behavior change* (2nd ed.). Guilford Press.

Heffner, M., Sperry, J., Eifert, G. H., & Detweiler, M. (2002). Acceptance and commitment therapy in the treatment of an adolescent female with anorexia nervosa: A case example. *Cognitive and Behavioral Practice, 9*(3), 232–236.

Hinds, E., Jones, L. B., Gau, J. M., Forrester, K. K., & Biglan, A. (2015). Teacher distress and the role of experiential avoidance. *Psychology in the Schools, 52*(3), 284–297.

Holland, M. L., Hawks, J., & Gimpel Peacock, G. (2017). *Emotional and behavioral problems of young children: Effective interventions in the preschool and kindergarten year* (2nd ed.). Guilford Press.

Hou, R. J., Wong, S. Y., Yip, B. H., Hung, A. T., Lo, H. H., Chan, P. H., Lo, C. S., Kwok, T. C., Tang, W. K., Mak, W. W., Mercer, S. W., & Ma, S. H. (2014). The effects of mindfulness-based stress reduction program on the mental health of family caregivers: A randomized controlled trial. *Psychotherapy and Psychosomatics, 83*(1), 45–53.

Iacona, J., & Johnson, S. (2018). Neurobiology of trauma and mindfulness for children. *Journal of Trauma Nursing, 25*(3), 187–191.

Jee, S. H., Couderc, J. P., Swanson, D., Gallegos, A., Hilliard, C., Blumkin, A., Cunningham, K., & Heinert, S. (2015). A pilot randomized trial teaching mindfulness-based stress reduction to traumatized youth in foster care. *Complementary Therapies in Clinical Practice, 21*(3), 201–209.

Jeffcoat, T., & Hayes, S. C. (2012). A randomized trial of ACT bibliotherapy on the mental health of K-12 teachers and staff. *Behaviour Research and Therapy, 50*(9), 571–579.

Jennings, P. A., Frank, J. L., Snowberg, K. E., Coccia, M. A., & Greenberg, M. T. (2013). Improving classroom learning environments by cultivating awareness and resilience in education (CARE): Results of a randomized controlled trial. *School Psychology Quarterly, 28*(4), 374–390.

Jensen, P., & Kenny, D. (2004). The effects of yoga on the attention and behavior of boys with attention-deficit/hyperactivity disorder (ADHD). *Journal of Attention Disorders, 7*(4), 205–216.

Jha, A., Krompinger, J., & Baime, M. (2007). Mindfulness training modifies subsystems of attention. *Cognitive, Affective and Behavioral Neuroscience, 7*(2), 109–119.

Kallapiran, K., Koo, S., Kirubakaran, R., & Hancock, K. (2015). Review: Effectiveness of mindfulness in improving mental health symptoms of children and adolescents: A meta-analysis. *Child and Adolescent Mental Health, 20*(4), 182–194.

Kerr, S. L., Lucas, L. J., DiDomenico, G. E., Mishra, V., Stanton, B. J., Shivde, G., Pero, A. N., Runyen, M. E., & Terry, G. M. (2017). Is mindfulness training useful for pre-service teachers? An exploratory investigation. *Teaching Education, 28*(4), 349–359.

Khoury, B., Lecomte, T., Fortin, G., Masse, M., Therien, P., Bouchard, V., Chapleau, M. A., Paquin, K., & Hofmann, S. G. (2013). Mindfulness-based therapy: A comprehensive meta-analysis. *Clinical Psychology Review, 33*(6), 763–771.

Khoury, B., Sharma, M., Rush, S. E., & Fournier, C. (2015). Mindfulness-based stress reduction for healthy individuals: A meta-analysis. *Journal of Psychosomatic Research, 78*(6), 519–528.

Klassen, R. M., & Chiu, M. M. (2010). Effects on teachers' self-efficacy and job satisfaction: Teacher gender, years of experience, and job stress. *Journal of Educational Psychology, 102*(3), 741–756.

Klatt, M., Browne, E., Harpster, K., & Case-Smith, J. (2012). P04.35. Sustained effects of a mindfulness-based classroom intervention on behavior in urban, underserved children. *BMC Complementary and Alternative Medicine, 12*(S1), 305.

Kuppusamy, M., Kamaldeen, D., Pitani, R., & Amaldas, J. (2016). Immediate effects of Bhramari Pranayama on resting cardiovascular parameters in healthy adolescents. *Journal of Clinical and Diagnostic Research, 10*, CC17–CC19.

Lazar, S. W., Bush, G., Gollub, R. L., Fricchione, G. L., Khalsa, G., & Benson, H. (2000). Functional brain mapping of the relaxation response and meditation. *NeuroReport: For Rapid Communication of Neuroscience Research, 11*(7), 1581–1585.

Leung, G. S. M., Yeung, K. C., & Wong, D. K. (2010). Academic stressors and anxiety in children: The role of paternal support. *Journal of Child and Family Studies, 19*(1), 90–100.

Liehr, P., & Diaz, N. (2010). A pilot student examining the effect of mindfulness on depression and anxiety for minority children. *Archives of Psychiatric Nursing, 24*(1), 69–71.

Livheim, F., Hayes, L., Ghaderi, A., Magnusdottir, T., Högfeldt, A., Rowse, J., Turner, S., Hayes, S. C., & Tengström, A. (2014). The effectiveness of acceptance and commitment therapy for adolescent mental health: Swedish and Australian pilot outcomes. *Journal of Child and Family Studies, 24*(4), 1016–1030.

Lloyd, J., Bond, F. W., & Flaxman, P. E. (2013). The value of psychological flexibility: Examining psychological mechanisms underpinning a cognitive behavioural therapy intervention for burnout. *Work & Stress, 27*(2), 181–199.

Lu, S., Huang, C., & Rios, J. (2017). Mindfulness and academic performance: An example of migrant children in China. *Children and Youth Services Review, 82*, 53–59.

Lucas-Thompson, R. G., Broderick, P. C., Coatsworth, J. D., & Smyth, J. M. (2019). New avenues for promoting mindfulness in adolescence using mHealth. *Journal of Child and Family Studies, 28*(1), 131–139.

Luoma, J. B., & Villatte, J. L. (2012). Mindfulness in the treatment of suicidal individuals. *Cognitive and Behavioral Practice, 9*(2), 265–276.

Ma, Y., She, Z., Siu, A. F., Zeng, X., & Liu, X. (2018). Effectiveness of online mindfulness-based interventions on psychological distress and the mediating role of emotion regulation. *Frontiers in Psychology, 9*, 2090.

MacDonell, K. W., & Prinz, R. J. (2017). A review of technology-based youth and family-focused interventions. *Clinical Child and Family Psychology Review, 20*(2), 185–200.

Malakouti, S. K., Rasouli, N., Rezaeian, M., Nojomi, M., Ghanbari, B., & Shahraki Mohammadi, A. (2020). Effectiveness of self-help mobile telephone applications (apps) for suicide prevention: A systematic review. *Medical journal of the Islamic Republic of Iran, 34*, 85.

Manuel, J. A., Somohano, V. C., & Bowen, S. (2017). Mindfulness practice and its relationship to the five-facet mindfulness questionnaire. *Mindfulness, 8*(2), 361–367.

Mathis, E., Shapiro, A., Hawkins, J. T., Charlot-Swilley, D., Lingo, K., Spencer, T., Trachtenberg, D., McPherson, S., Domitrovich, C., & Biel, M. G. (2018). 1.40 Cultivating mindfulness in parents of young children: Effects of a mindful parenting intervention pilot in a low-income community. *Journal of the American Academy of Child & Adolescent Psychiatry, 57*(10), S148.

Mendelson, T., Greenberg, M. T., Dariotis, J. K., Gould, L. F., Rhoades, B. L., & Leaf, P. J. (2010). Feasibility and preliminary outcomes of a school-based mindfulness intervention for urban youth. *Journal of Abnormal Child Psychology, 38*(7), 985–994.

Metz, S. M., Frank, J. L., Reibel, D., Cantrell, T., Sanders, R., & Broderick, P. C. (2013). The effectiveness of the learning to BREATHE program on adolescent emotion regulation. *Research in Human Development, 10*(3), 252–272.

Mindful Schools. (2015a). *Mindfulness fundamentals.* www.mindfulschools.org/training/mindfulness-fundamentals/

Moody, K., Abrahams, B., Baker, R., Santizo, R., Manwani, D., Carullo, V., Eugenio, D., & Carroll, A. (2017). A randomized trial of yoga for children hospitalized with sickle cell vaso-occlusive crisis. *Journal of Pain and Symptom Management, 53*(6), 1026–1034.

Mrazek, M. D., Franklin, M. S., Phillips, D., Baird, B., & Schooler, J. W. (2013). Mindfulness training improves working memory capacity and GRE performance while reducing mind wandering. *Psychological Science, 24*(5), 776–778.

Napoli, M., Krech, P. R., & Holley, L. C. (2005). Mindfulness training for elementary school students: The Attention Academy. *Journal of Applied School Psychology, 21*(1), 99–125.

National Center for Complementary and Integrative Medicine. (2017). *Meditation: In depth.* NCCIH. www.nccih.nih.gov/health/meditation-in-depth

National Center for Education Statistics (2015, November). *Teacher turnover: Stayers, movers, and leavers.* NCES. https://nces.ed.gov/programs/coe/indicator_slc.asp

National Commission on Teaching and America's Future. (2007). *The high cost of teacher turnover* [Policy brief]. NCTAF. ERIC. https://eric.ed.gov/?id=ED498001

Neece, C. L. (2013). Mindfulness-based stress reduction for parents of young children with developmental delays: Implications for parental mental health and child behavior problems. *Journal of Applied Research in Intellectual Disabilities, 27*(2), 174–186.

Noggle, J. J., Steiner, N. J., Minami, T., & Khalsa, S. B. (2012). Benefits of yoga for psychosocial well-being in a us high school curriculum: A preliminary randomized controlled trial. *Journal of Developmental and Behavioral Pediatrics, 33,* 193–201.

Oberle, E., Schonert-Reichl, K. A., Lawlor, M. S., & Thomson, K. C. (2012). Mindfulness and inhibitory control in early adolescence. *The Journal of Early Adolescence, 32*(4), 565–588.

O'Brien, K. M., Larson, C. M., & Murrell, A. R. (2008). Third-wave behavior therapies for children and adolescents: Progress, challenges and future directions. In L. A. Greco & S. C. Hayes (Eds.), *Acceptance & mindfulness treatments for children and adolescents: A practitioner's guide* (pp. 15–35). New Harbinger Publications.

Poddar, S., Sinha, V. K., & Urbi, M. (2015). Acceptance and commitment therapy on parents of children and adolescents with autism spectrum disorders. *International Journal of Educational and Psychological Researches, 1*(3), 221–225.

Querstret, D., & Cropley, M. (2013). Assessing treatments used to reduce rumination and/or worry: A systematic review. *Clinical Psychology Review, 33*(8), 996–1009.

Raes, F., Griffith, J. W., Van der Gucht, K., & Williams, J. M. G. (2014). School-based prevention and reduction of depression in adolescents: A cluster-randomized controlled trial of a mindfulness group program. *Mindfulness, 5*(5), 477–486.

Razza, R. A., Bergen-Cico, D., & Raymond, K. (2015). Enhancing preschoolers' self-regulation via mindful yoga. *Journal of Child and Family Studies, 24*(2), 372–385.

Roeser, R. W., Schonert-Reichl, K. A., Jha, A., Cullen, M., Wallace, L., Wilensky, R., Oberle, E., Thomson, K., Taylor, C., & Harrison, J. (2013). Mindfulness training and reductions in teacher stress and burnout: Results from two randomized, waitlist-control field trials. *Journal of Educational Psychology, 105*(3), 787–804.

Roodenrys, S., Badawi, A., & Lovegrove, W. (2017). How strong is the evidence that mindfulness produces healthy psychological changes in children? In T. Ditrich, R. Wiles, & B. Lovegrove (Eds.), *Mindfulness and education: Research and practice* (pp. 33–54). Cambridge Scholars Publishing.

Sanada, K., Montero-Marin, J., Alda Díez, M., Salas-Valero, M., Pérez-Yus, M. C., Morillo, H., Demarzo, M. M., García-Toro, M., & García-Campayo, J. (2016). Effects of mindfulness-based interventions on salivary cortisol in healthy adults: A meta-analytical review. *Frontiers in Physiology, 7,* 471.

Schechter, J. C., Brennan, P. A., Cunningham, P. B., Foster, S. L., & Whitmore, E. (2012). Stress, cortisol, and externalizing behavior in adolescent males: An examination in the context of multisystemic therapy. *Journal of Abnormal Child Psychology, 40,* 913–922.

Schonert-Reichl, K. A., & Lawlor, M. S. (2010). The effects of a mindfulness-based education program on pre- and early adolescents' well-being and social and emotional competence. *Mindfulness, 1*(3), 137–151.

Schonert-Reichl, K. A., Oberle, E., Lawlor, M. S., Abbot, D., Thomson, K., Oberlander, T., & Diamond, A. (2015). Enhancing cognitive and social-emotional development through a simple-to-administer mindfulness-based school program for elementary school children: A randomized controlled trial. *Developmental Psychology, 51*(1), 52–66.

Sedlmeier, P., Eberth, J., Schwarz, M., Zimmermann, D., Haarig, F., Jaeger, S., & Kunze, S. (2012). The psychological effects of meditation: A meta-analysis. *Psychological Bulletin, 138*(6), 1139–1171.

Semple, R. J., Lee, J., Rosa, D., & Miller, L. F. (2010). A randomized trial of mindfulness-based cognitive therapy for children: Promoting mindful attention to enhance social-emotional resiliency in children. *Journal of Child and Family Studies, 19*(2), 218–229.

Seney, R. W., & Mishou, M. A. (2018). The importance of mindfulness training for teachers. *Gifted Education International, 34*(2), 155–161.

Sharp Donahoo, L., Siegrist, B., & Garrett-Wright, D. (2018). Addressing compassion fatigue and stress of special education teachers and professional staff using mindfulness and prayer. *The Journal of School Nursing, 34*(6), 442–448.

Sibinga, E. M., Perry-Parrish, C., Chung, S. E., Johnson, S. B., Smith, M., & Ellen, J. M. (2013). School-based mindfulness instruction for urban male youth: A small randomized controlled trial. *Preventive Medicine, 57*(6), 799–801.

Sibinga, E. M., Webb, L., Ghazarian, S. R., & Ellen J. M. (2016). School-based mindfulness instruction: An RCT. *Pediatrics, 137*(1), 2015–2532.

Singh, N. N., Lancioni, G. E., Winton, A. S. W., Fisher, B. C., Wahler, R. G., McAleavey, K., Singh, J., & Sabaawi, M. (2006). Mindful parenting decreases aggression, noncompliance, and self-injury in children with autism. *Journal of Emotional and Behavioral Disorders, 14*(3), 169–177.

Singh, N. N., Lancioni, G. E., Winton, A. S. W., Karazsia, B. T., & Singh, J. (2013). Mindfulness training for teachers changes the behavior of their preschool students. *Research in Human Development, 10*(3), 211–233.

Stueck, M., & Gloeckner, N. (2005). Yoga for children in the mirror of the science: Working spectrum and practice fields of the training of relaxation with elements of yoga for children. *Early Child Development and Care, 175*(4), 371–377.

Taylor, C., Harrison, J., Haimovitz, K., Oberle, E., Thomson, K., Schonert-Reichl, K., & Roeser, R. W. (2016). Examining ways that a mindfulness-based intervention reduces stress in public school teachers: A mixed-methods study. *Mindfulness, 7*(6), 1449.

Taylor, L., & Adelman, H. S. (2001). Enlisting appropriate parental cooperation and involvement in children's mental health treatment. In E. R. Welfel & R. E. Ingersoll (Eds.), *The mental health desk reference* (pp. 219–224). Wiley.

Telles, S., Gupta, R. K., Gandharva, K., Vishwakarma, B., Kala, N., & Balkrishna, A. (2019). Immediate effect of a yoga breathing practice on attention and anxiety in pre-teen children. *Children (Basel, Switzerland), 6*(7), 84.

Tracey, D., Gray, T., Truong, S., & Ward, K. (2018). Combining acceptance and commitment therapy with adventure therapy to promote psychological wellbeing for children at-risk. *Frontiers in Psychology, 9*, 1565.

Van Dam, N. T., Earleywine, M., & Borders, A. (2010). Measuring mindfulness? An item response theory analysis of the mindful attention awareness scale. *Personality and Individual Differences, 49*(7), 805–810.

Van Dam, N. T., van Vugt, M. K., Vago, D. R., Schmalzl, L., Saron, C. D., Olendzki, A., Meissner, T., Lazar, S. W., Kerr, C. E., Gorchov, J., Fox, K. C. R., Field, B. A., Britton, W. B., Brefczynski-Lewis, J. A., & Meyer, D. E. (2018). Mind the hype: A critical evaluation and prescriptive agenda for research on mindfulness and meditation. *Perspectives on Psychological Science, 13*(1), 36–61.

van de Weijer-Bergsma, E., Formsma, A. R., de Bruin, E. I., & Bogels, S. M. (2012). The effectiveness of mindfulness training on behavioral problems and attentional functioning in adolescents with ADHD. *Journal of Child and Family Studies, 21*(5), 775–787.

Viglas, M., & Perlman, M. (2018). Effects of a mindfulness-based program on young children's self-regulation, prosocial behavior and hyperactivity. *Journal of Child and Family Studies, 27*(4), 1150–1161.

Vøllestad, J., Nielsen, M. B., & Nielsen, G. H. (2012). Mindfulness- and acceptance-based interventions for anxiety disorders: A systematic review and meta-analysis. *British Journal of Clinical Psychology, 51*(3), 239–260.

Walker, J., & Pacik, D. (2017). Controlled rhythmic yogic breathing as complementary treatment for post-traumatic stress disorder in military veterans: A case series. *Medical Acupuncture, 29*(3), 232–238.

Wall, R. (2005). Tai chi and mindfulness-based stress reduction in a Boston public middle school. *Journal of Pediatric Health Care, 19*(4), 230–237.

Whittingham, K., Sanders, M., McKinlay, L., & Boyd, R. (2016). Parenting intervention combined with acceptance and commitment therapy: A trial with families of children with cerebral palsy. *Journal of Pediatric Psychology, 41*(5), 531–542.

Wicksell, R. K., Melin, L., & Olsson, G. L. (2007). Exposure and acceptance in the rehabilitation of adolescents with idiopathic chronic pain – A pilot study. *European Journal of Pain, 11*(3), 267–274.

Wicksell, R. K., Olsson, G. L., & Hayes, S. C. (2011). Mediators of change in acceptance and commitment therapy for pediatric chronic pain. *Pain, 152*(12), 2792–2801.

Wright, S., Day, A., & Howells, K. (2009). Mindfulness and the treatment of anger problems. *Aggression and Violent Behavior, 14*(5), 396–401.

Zelano, C., Jiang, H., Zhou, G., Arora, N., Schuele, S., Rosenow, J., & Gottfried, J. A. (2016). Nasal respiration entrains human limbic oscillations and modulates cognitive function. *Journal of Neuroscience, 36*(49), 12448–12467.

Zelazo, P. D., & Lyons, K. E. (2012). Mindfulness training in childhood. *Human Development, 54*(2), 61–65.

Zenner, C., Herrnleben-Kurz, S., & Walach, H. (2014). Mindfulness-based interventions in schools-a systematic review and meta-analysis. *Frontiers in Psychiatry, 5*, 603.

Zoogman, S., Goldberg, S. B., Hoyt, W. T., & Miller, L. (2015). Mindfulness interventions with youth: A meta-analysis. *Mindfulness, 6*(2), 290–302.

3 Mindfulness Techniques for Individual Work

> **Roadmap to Chapter 3:**
> This chapter will prepare you to implement mindfulness with individual students. We'll explore mindfulness practice in five areas:
>
> - Breathwork
> - Body Scan
> - Meditation
> - Heartfulness and gratitude
> - Yoga and other physical practices

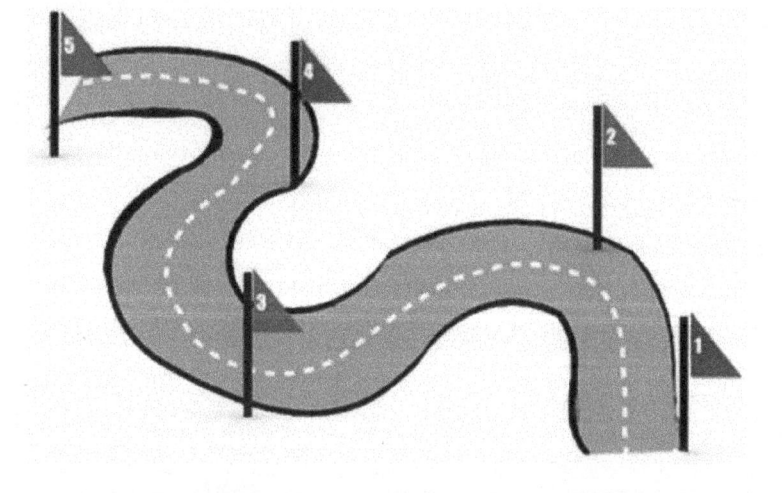

Mindfulness has become a common practice in individual counseling with youth (Zelazo & Lyons, 2012), and, more recently, in school-based mental health services (Renshaw & Cook, 2017). As outlined in Chapter 2, research supports mindfulness practice as a Tier 3 intervention.

DOI: 10.4324/9781003318101-3

This chapter explores mindfulness practices that can be used individually with youth in the schools. Table 3.1 provides an overview of the mindfulness strategies that we will explore. We will begin with breathwork, which is the cornerstone of most mindfulness practices. Next, we will describe how to engage youth in a body scan exercise. Meditation and other mindfulness techniques, such as gratitude practices and yoga, are then presented. The chapter offers practitioner prompts and scripts, along with examples of the use and adaption of specific techniques for younger children. As a reminder, Jennings (2015) suggests practitioners regularly use these skills in their personal lives, as this will increase the effectiveness of teaching these skills to youth. Chapters 5 and 6 will look at how these practices can be used with small groups, as well as how they can be adapted for use in classroom and school-wide programming.

Figure 3.1 is a flow chart for how to choose a mindfulness technique given common presenting concerns. Of course, the mindfulness techniques you select will vary dependent upon multiple factors, such as the youth's age, developmental level, specific needs and concerns, and personal background.

Introducing Mindfulness to Children

When first introducing mindfulness to youth, it can be helpful to begin by asking them if they have ever heard of the concept of mindfulness, and if so, what they know about it. This helps you gauge the starting point for the child's practice. Through this discussion, you can also address any misconceptions about mindfulness (Rechtschaffen, 2016). For example, a common misconception is that to be mindful means to be completely without thought, or that you must be engaging in a formal meditation practice in order to be mindful. You can then introduce the definition of mindfulness. For older youth, a common definition of mindfulness is paying attention in a nonjudgmental way to the present moment (Kabat-Zinn, 2003). For younger children, you can simplify the description as noticing what is happening around you and inside you (both in your mind and in your body). Following this introduction, it is recommended that you provide brief psychoeducation about how mindfulness can help their minds and bodies, as this will increase the likelihood that they will practice and use these techniques.

Educating Youth on How Stress and Mindfulness Affects the Body

Supporting students in understanding how their brains and bodies respond to stress can be empowering, particularly as you highlight how mindfulness practices can counteract these effects. It also helps to normalize that their reactions to stress are common, reducing possible feelings of isolation and shame. In their book *Buddha's Brain* (2009),

Table 3.1 Summary of mindfulness-based strategies in this chapter.

Strategies	Definitions	Expected Time	Age Range/Adaptations	Target Process/Outcome
Diaphragmatic Breathing	Breathing in through the diaphragm aids the lungs in fully expanding with air and breathing out allows the muscle fibers of the diaphragm to relax (aiding the relaxation response). Different poses, such as crocodile, relaxation, seated or standing posture, can assist in this form of breathing.	Varies	Age 3 and older	Aids in the relaxation response, slows SNS arousal, sets the foundation for meditation, yoga, and other mindfulness techniques.
4x8 Breathing	Breathing in to the count of 4, breathing out to the count of 8. Elongated exhales are linked to the relaxation response.	Varies	Age 3 and older, with adaptations in length of outbreath (perhaps 3x6)	Aids in the relaxation response, slows SNS arousal, sets the foundation for meditation, yoga, and other mindfulness techniques.
Alternate Nostril Breathing	Closing off one nostril at a time during inhalation and exhalation. Helpful in reducing sympathetic nervous system activation.	3 + minutes	Age 10 and older	Reduces SNS activation. More helpful in reducing blood pressure levels than other forms of breathwork.
Progressive Muscle Relaxation	Different muscle groups are systematically tightened and released, often coupled with deep breathing.	5+ minutes	Age 3 and older, with script adaptation as noted	Reduces physical tension and anxiety. Works well with youth experiencing anxiety, stress, or somatic complaints.
Focused Meditation	The practice of focused attention involves intentionally directing and maintaining attention toward a target.	Varies	Age 3 and older, with adaptations as noted	This basic mindfulness practice helps to settle and focus the mind on a specific target. Works well for any presenting concern wherein thoughts are problematic.

Open Awareness Meditation	Remaining aware of our surroundings and observing things happening without getting caught up in thoughts or judgments.	Varies	Age 7 and older	This basic mindfulness practice helps to settle and focus the mind on the present moment. Works well for any presenting concern wherein thoughts are problematic.
Specific Mindfulness Practices: Mindful Eating/ Mindful Walking	Mindful eating is paying attention to food using all five senses, moment by moment, without judgment. Mindful walking is a way to practice moving without a goal or intention.	5 minutes	Age 3 and older	Tangible practices geared toward increasing mindful awareness. Suited for anyone practicing mindfulness.
Gratitude and Heartfulness	The act of focusing on what we are grateful for, along with increasing our desire to bond and connect with others and the world (heartfulness) has been shown to be linked to positive emotional well-being.	Varies	Age 3 and older, with adaptations as noted	Increases focus on the positive, thereby increasing well-being. Works well with all ages in increasing empathy and general good mood.
Yoga	Coordinating breathwork, meditation, and specific postures to focus and calm the mind.	Varies	Age 3 and older, with adaptations as noted	Can reduce anxiety and aggression and increase mental well-being in youth.

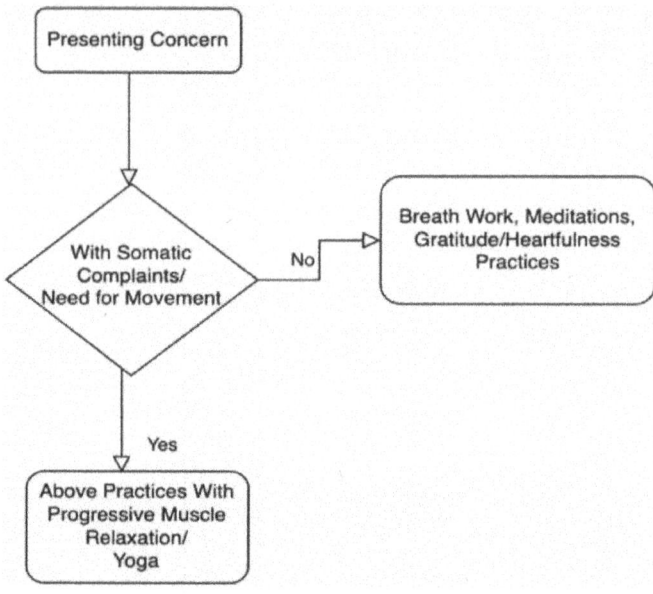

Figure 3.1 Flow Chart for Choosing Mindfulness Techniques.

Hanson and Mendius discuss how our brains have adapted over time to more readily attend to and respond to negative information. They introduce this idea through "sticks" and "carrots." When explaining this to youth, describe how "sticks" are things that feel threatening or unpleasant and activate our sympathetic nervous system (SNS; the fight, flee, or freeze response) and "carrots" are things we desire and are pleasant and activate our parasympathetic nervous system (PNS), which initiates a rest and relaxation response.

In general, we have evolved to pay greater attention to the unpleasant or negative experiences (the sticks) over the carrots in order to survive. This "negativity bias" highlights the bad news, overlooks the good news, and creates uncomfortable feeling states, such as anxiety and depression (Hanson & Mendius, 2009). Our ancestors had to pay attention to the snapping of twigs in the forest (e.g., that may indicate a tiger is stalking us) in order to survive. If we did not protect ourselves, we would have become extinct. The challenge, however, is that today our thoughts can trigger our SNS response as real threats, even when there is no actual threat present (Smith, 2011).

The other challenge is that once a particular carrot, or goal, is attained, we often trick ourselves and quickly replace it with another carrot that we are striving toward, leaving us unable to enjoy the completion of the original goal. For example, a high achieving teen may devote significant effort and attention toward excelling on their final exams. At the end of the semester, the carrot is quickly replaced, and the teen immediately shifts focus toward achieving other accomplishments, not allowing themselves to celebrate in the successes they just achieved. All the while, days, months, and even years may go by, all lived stressfully and unsatisfied, as the teen never feels they have accomplished their desired results.

Once you have provided psychoeducation about the negativity bias and how our bodies respond to stress, emphasize how mindfulness can help to deactivate the stress response, and consequently, allow our minds to see things more objectively and more positively. By training our bodies and our minds to attend more purposefully to our internal and external experiences, we can, in turn, reduce emotional distress and suffering. This conversation helps students understand that they do have control of their responses to their thoughts and feelings, resulting in an increased sense of self-efficacy. A sample script is provided below:

PRACTITIONER: *We are going to talk about "sticks" and "carrots" today. "Sticks" are things that feel threatening or upsetting. They create a response that releases chemicals in our bodies that speed up our heart rate and raise our blood pressure, which prepares us to fight, run away, or stay still in order to protect ourselves. Getting in a fight with a friend, getting in trouble with a teacher, or failing a test are examples of sticks we usually want to avoid. "Carrots" are things we want and that feel good. Carrots release chemicals in our bodies that feel pleasurable and rewarding. Getting a good grade, getting a compliment, or winning a game would all likely make us feel good, making us want to do those things again.*

In general, we pay more attention to the negative stuff, or the sticks, over the carrots, the good stuff, in order to survive. This "negativity bias" highlights the bad news, overlooks the good news, and can lead us to feel sad or scared. Thousands of years ago in order to survive we needed to pay greater attention to threats around us, like the snapping of twigs in the forest, which could mean a tiger is after us. If we did not protect ourselves, we could have been hurt, or worse! We don't usually have tigers after us anymore, but our thoughts can act like tigers. They jump out at us in our minds and feel like real threats.

Mindfulness can help to turn down the stress response and allow our minds to see things more clearly and more positively. It can help us focus on the present moment to help us find ways to feel better now. In this way, we change our reactions to our thoughts and feelings, which can help us to feel calmer and more in control.

The practitioner can also explain to a youth the idea of how we often put off our well-being, and how mindfulness can help us focus on using the "now" to take care of ourselves.

PRACTITIONER: *The other challenge is that we often replace the carrots that are in front of us with different, bigger, or more satisfying future carrots. Once we have reached a particular carrot, or goal, we often trick ourselves by not enjoying completing the first goal and quickly replacing it with another carrot that we work toward. For example, a student may focus all of their energy into doing really well on final exams. However, once they complete their final exams and are assigned good grades, they may immediately shift their focus to extensively practicing a sport, rather than taking some time to appreciate and celebrate in their academic accomplishments. All the while, we may spend days, months, and even years all lived stressfully. And because we do this, we may never feel that we have reached our goal. Mindfulness can help to focus on the present moment and find ways to help us feel better now.*

In addition to the above scripts, an experiential introduction can help with understanding the concept of mindfulness. There are several ways to introduce youth to mindfulness experientially, including through breathwork and paying attention to their body or their surroundings. Modeling is one of the best forms of learning for youth, and we recommend you model the skills for the child first, then practice the skill with the child and provide feedback.

Breathwork

We begin with breathwork, as it is often considered the foundation of mindfulness. Connection to breath aids focused attention and experiential awareness (the essence of mindfulness). No matter what mindfulness or meditation strategy is being taught, or the age of the student with whom you are working, breathwork is almost always incorporated. Breath plays a powerful role in our ability to calm the body and mind and increase conscious awareness of the present moment. Rapid breathing, particularly through the nose with increased inhalation versus exhalation, leads to the experience of anxiety, and even panic (Zelano et al., 2016). Yogic breath, with deep controlled inhalations and exhalations, can help to reduce anxious symptoms (Walker & Pacik, 2017). Slowed breath is implicated in the relaxation response. It is thought to activate the PNS and decrease activation of the fight, flight, freeze response, or SNS (Asmundson & Stein, 1994; Elliott, 2010). Giving the youth an age-appropriate understanding of the SNS and PNS response can help gain buy-in for doing breathwork. Mindful breath is the vehicle by which students can emerge from the thinking mind and come back into the present moment. As Hanh (2012) wrote, "The moment you begin to practice mindful breathing, your body and your mind begin to come back together. . . . And every one of us can do it, even a child" (pg. 57).

There are various practices associated with mindfulness and breathwork. Three of the most common practices are: diaphragmatic breathing, 4x8 breathing, and alternate nostril breathing (ANB). Handouts for the practitioner are provided for each of these techniques. To introduce breathwork to youth, the practitioner can adapt the following script to meet the needs of the youth's age, modifying with simpler or more sophisticated language as appropriate.

PRACTITIONER: *Today we are going to be focusing on how we breathe; this is important because when we are under stress or feel upset, we often hold our breath or breathe very quickly. This can make us feel even more uncomfortable.*

Diaphragmatic Breathing
Ages: 3 and older
Time: varies

Diaphragmatic breathing is the starting point for any student doing breathwork. The diaphragm is a dome-shaped muscle located in the torso under the rib cage. Breathing in through the diaphragm helps the lungs fully expand with air; breathing out allows the muscle in the diaphragm to relax (aiding the relaxation response). Breathing primarily with the chest muscles arouses the SNS, creating tension; breathing through the diaphragm increases parasympathetic activity, increasing relaxation (Elliott, 2010). In the practice of mindfulness, meditation, and relaxation, diaphragmatic breathing is critical. Slowing down the number of breaths taken per minute is associated with increased relaxation. Research supports the fact that SNS activity reduces when subjects breathe slowly (Oneda et al., 2010; Zelano et al., 2016). Most mindful breathing techniques recommend slow diaphragmatic breaths. With older or more developmentally mature youth, the above rationale for the use of diaphragmatic breathing can secure further buy-in. There are various ways to help youth practice diaphragmatic breathing. Forms 3.1 to 3.4 include descriptions and diagrams for crocodile pose, relaxation pose, and seated or standing posture. Each of these poses are discussed in Table 3.2.

In each of the following poses, encourage the youth to pay attention to their breathing. Model for them how to take in deep, slow breaths, in and out through their nose or, alternatively, in through the nose and out through the mouth. Breathing through the nose has been found to drop blood pressure, heart rate, and increase carbon dioxide, leading to the relaxation response (Nestor, 2020). When we inhale, our heart rate speeds up, but when we exhale, it slows down. Elongating the exhale can help with reducing depression and anxiety, enhance relaxation, and improve lung capacity (Nestor, 2020; Seppala et al., 2020). Discussing with older youth (late elementary age and older) the benefits of this form of deep breathing can help them in understanding why they are using it and may encourage them to therefore use it more. The metaphor of

Table 3.2 Summary of breath poses.

Strategies	Definitions
Crocodile Pose	This pose entails laying prone on the stomach, with arms folded at about a 45-degree angle above the shoulders.
Relaxation Pose	The youth lies flat on their back with their arms and legs slightly spread.
Seated Posture	The youth is seated in a chair, with erect spine and feet flat on the floor.
Standing Posture	The youth is standing up, arms at the side, feet firmly planted on the floor with tall spine.

breath as an anchor can also be useful (Germer, 2009). Suggest that the youth is the boat, their thoughts are the waves, and their breath is the anchor. When thoughts pull us "out to sea," we can use the breath to anchor us back mindfully to the present moment.

Crocodile Pose: The best physical posture for initially practicing diaphragmatic breathing is crocodile pose. This is because, in this position, the diaphragm begins to assist breathing naturally. This pose entails laying prone on the stomach, with arms folded at about a 45-degree angle above the shoulders. If that's uncomfortable, they may prop their upper body with a thin pillow or a blanket, draping their chin over the prop. Form 3.1 contains directions and a picture for this posture. Once the youth has tried this pose, or if they are not comfortable in this pose, you may move on to the other poses listed below.

Relaxation Pose: A simple version of diaphragmatic breathing is relaxation pose, also known as shavasana. In this posture, the individual lies flat on their back with their arms and legs slightly spread. The navel region in this position rises with each inhalation and falls with each exhalation. For young children, it can be helpful to place an object, such as a stuffed animal, on the abdomen in order for them to see the rise and fall of the object with each breath. See Form 3.2 for directions and a picture of this posture.

Seated or Standing Posture: Seated posture is just as it sounds: the youth is seated in a chair, with erect spine and feet flat on the floor. Seated posture, coupled with breathwork, should be practiced regularly with youth, as students often find themselves in seated poses in classroom settings (see Form 3.3). Standing posture is also known as mountain pose. This is a position wherein the child is standing up, arms at the side, feet firmly planted on the floor with tall spine (see Form 3.4).

4x8 Breathing.
Ages: 3 and older with adaptation
Time: Varies

Once the youth has mastered diaphragmatic breath and basic poses, the next practice, 4x8 breathing, also known as 2:1 breathing, builds on these skills. In 4x8 breathing, the exhalation of the breath is twice as long as the inhalation. Exhalation has been linked to the relaxation response (Zelano et al., 2016). This form of breathing helps to further regulate the motion of the lungs, helping to facilitate relaxation to aid in mindful awareness (Clark, 2019). When one is in an anxious or panicked state, the breathing rhythm becomes more rapid, leading to more time inhaling than exhaling. 4x8 breathing has been found to have both mental and physical benefits, including altering the activation of the nervous system and managing blood pressure and hypertension (Adhana et al., 2013). Controlled 4x8 breaths can help to modulate the nervous system response when used during relaxation or meditative states.

The instructions for completing 4x8 breathing are simple and described in the following script.

PRACTITIONER: *Today we are going to try a type of breathing called 4 by 8 breathing. What this means is we are going to be taking deep, diaphragmatic breaths in to the count of 4, hold it briefly at the top, and let it out to the count of 8. In this way, we are breathing out twice as long as we are breathing in. We do this because it helps to calm our bodies and our minds faster than our usual way of breathing. Let's try it together.*

Child breathes in as practitioner slowly counts 1-2-3-4, pauses at the top, then counts slowly out 1-2-3-4-5-6-7-8.

Age adaptations for breathwork: Note that a more sophisticated or detailed explanation for the physiological effects of 4x8 breaths can be offered to older youth or those curious about the effects of breath on their mental state. For younger children this pace can be shortened to 2x4 or 3x6 breaths. The rate of the counting can also be adjusted faster or slower, depending on the development of the child or if the practitioner notes that the child is struggling with this form of breathing in the beginning. If the child has challenges with nose breathing (e.g., has a cold) or breathing out through their mouth, these too can be altered so the child is more comfortable (e.g., have the child only breathe through their nose or mouth). Other strategies for younger children to help them with 4x8 breathing is using a prop, such as a pinwheel or blowing bubbles. These two props can help focus on a deep inhalation through the nose, then a more elongated exhale through the mouth. The longer, smoother and more controlled the exhale, the longer the pinwheel will spin, or the more bubbles will be blown. You can also encourage the child to pretend they are smelling flowers (deep breath in through nose) and then blowing out birthday candles (elongated breath though the mouth).

With adaptation, diaphragmatic and 4x8 breathing can be used successfully across age levels. The third practice of ANB, a more complex breathing technique, will be discussed next.

Alternate Nostril Breathing
Ages: 10 years and older
Time: 3+ minutes

ANB has been found effective in reducing SNS activation and may be more effective in reducing blood pressure levels than other forms of breathwork (Telles et al., 2014). A study by Sinha and colleagues (2013), found that with 15 minutes a day for 6 weeks of ANB training, the relaxation response was enhanced significantly. Related research found that during ANB there was a significant decrease in systolic blood pressure and respiration rate in participants as compared to controls (Telles et al., 2014).

When using this breathing technique, begin in a seated comfortable posture. With the right hand, briefly close off both nostrils, then open the left nostril and slowly inhale. Close the left nostril and open the right nostril to slowly exhale. With the right nostril still open, slowly inhale. Then close the right and open the left to exhale. Continue alternating nostrils.

ANB can be particularly helpful for youth who have significant physiological symptoms (e.g., accelerated heart rate, high blood pressure) of stress and anxiety. ANB can be used with older youth (late elementary–high school students) and adults. It may be too complex motorically for younger children. Form 3.5 contains directions and an illustration of the practice of ANB. Other techniques, such as 4x8 breathing and body scanning, are more appropriate for younger youth.

How to Choose Which Breathing Technique to Use

Diaphragmatic breathing is the start of most mindfulness techniques. Encouraging youth to use the different poses as they breathe is key to being able to successfully progress in their mindfulness practice. Both 4x8 breathwork and ANB are helpful in calming the SNS and reducing the stress response. While 4x8 breaths can be used with almost any youth for any presenting concern, the more complicated ANB is typically reserved for older youth who have significant physical symptoms of anxiety and stress, such as high blood pressure and rapid heart rate. For children of almost any age, breathwork can be combined with body scanning, which is described next.

Body Scan Meditation
Ages: 3 and older with adaptation
Time: 5+ minutes

Body scan meditation is an exercise where you purposefully bring your attention to your body, noticing the different sensations, as you mentally scan from your head to your toes. This exercise is often coupled with breathwork. When we become anxious or stressed, our muscles often tighten, which can lead to physical ailments such as backaches, headaches, stomachaches, and the like. Because children tend to be more somatic when upset, body scanning can be a particularly appropriate intervention. Oftentimes, we fail to appreciate that our physical sensations are connected to our emotional state. When conducting a body scan, we purposefully check in with our bodies and bring our full attention to the present moment and whatever bodily sensations are occurring, without judgment or efforts to change these experiences. A sample script is offered in Form 3.6. Before beginning this exercise, the child should be comfortably sitting in a chair and using 4x8 breaths. As with many of the other techniques offered in this book, it is best if the practitioner first models this technique and then does the exercise along with the child. Below is an excerpt from the sample script.

PRACTITIONER: *Good, now we are going to shift our focus to our hands. Notice where your hands are currently located. Are they in your lap, holding onto the chair, or clasped together? Are they feeling cold or warm; tense or relaxed? No need to move them or do anything with them. Just take a moment to notice them.*

Once you have prompted the youth to check in with the different parts of their body, scanning from head to toe, spend the final few minutes coaching the youth to continue engaging in diaphragmatic breathing.

Meditation Techniques

Once the student has practiced breathwork, meditation techniques can be combined with breathing practices in order to address thoughts that may be contributing to the youth's presenting concerns. Meditation is the formal practice of purposefully guiding your mind toward a particular anchor. When thoughts wander, youth are coached to simply notice this and gently guide their focus back to their anchor. Meditation relates to, but is not interchangeable with, the concept of mindfulness. Mindfulness is simply the act of paying attention to the present moment and can be informally incorporated into daily living, as well as formally integrated into meditative practice. Meditation practices teach us how to settle our minds. When we ruminate on or fuse to our thoughts, we become distracted and mindless, often leading to unproductive emotional states, such as anxiety, depression, or anger. Meditation, however, allows us to focus our attention, which helps to decrease ruminative thinking. In this section, two types of meditative techniques will be described: focused attention and open awareness.

Focused Attention Meditation
Ages: 3 and older with adaptations
Time: Varies

The practice of focused attention meditation involves intentionally directing and maintaining attention on a target. The target for focused attention can either be external (e.g., an object in the room) or internal (e.g., breath or the soles of the feet). For younger children, it is often easiest to begin with an external focus since that is less abstract, as described next.

External Focus. An external object is best for directing focus when it is stable and consistent. Objects that are not stable (e.g., a television show, an animal, another person) can be too distracting. Examples of objects for the youth to focus on externally could include the following:

• A candle – watching the flame
• A sound – listening to a gong or chime
• A plant or other object – fixing one's gaze on the item

An example of how an external object would be used in meditation is outlined in the following script:

PRACTITIONER: *Now that we have practiced our diaphragmatic breaths, we are going to focus our attention on our breath. We will start by sitting up in our chairs, with our feet flat on the floor and our hands in our laps.*
   Model this for the youth.
PRACTITIONER: *Good, now we are going to focus on relaxing our face as we breathe through our nose, in to the count of 4, and out to the count of 8. With each breath in and out, notice your cheeks soften, your jaw and forehead relax.*
   Model 4x8 breaths for the youth.
PRACTITIONER: *Now, as we are taking our deep, 4x8 breaths, we are going to put our attention on the candle in front of us and watch its flame. (pause) Notice how the colors are different at the top of the flame than the bottom. (pause) Notice how the flame flickers, almost like it is dancing. When a thought comes into your mind, just allow that thought to leave your mind and bring your attention back on the candle and your deep, 4x8 breaths.*
   Pause here and allow time for the youth to engage in deep breathing and observe the candle.
PRACTITIONER: *Good. Let's take one more deep breath in, and out. Slowly we will return our awareness back into the room.*

Internal Focus. There are many ways to help youth obtain a sense of internal focused attention. Examples for internal focus could include:

- Visualization – picturing a peaceful place or image in one's mind
- A mantra – repeating a grounding word, phrase, or sound in one's mind
- A part of the body – focusing on a particular sensation or area of the body, such as the feet
- Breath – noticing the rise and fall of the abdomen

Below is a script primarily centered on the breath.

PRACTITIONER: *Now that we have practiced our diaphragmatic breaths, we are going to focus our attention on our breath. We will start by sitting up in our chairs, with our feet flat on the floor and our hands in our laps.*

Model this for the youth.

PRACTITIONER: *Imagine your spine is held by a thread coming from the top of your head and attached to the ceiling.*

Model an erect, yet not stiff posture for the youth.

PRACTITIONER: *Good, now we are going to focus on relaxing our faces as we breathe through our nose, in to the count of 4, and out to the count of 8. With each breath in and out, notice your cheeks soften, your jaw and forehead relax. Go ahead and either close your eyes, if you are comfortable with that, or soften your gaze so you are not looking at anything in particular.*

Model for the youth a relaxed facial expression and 4x8 breaths, with closed eyes.

PRACTITIONER: *Good. If you become distracted by something else in the room, or if your mind wanders, bring your attention back to your breath once you realize you have lost focus. (pause) Notice how your stomach rises and falls with each deep breath, in and out. Focus right now just on your breath and the sound of my voice. Taking a deep breath in to the count of 4 through your nose (pause), and out to the count of 8.*

Model for the youth a minute of deep breathing, with feet flat on the floor, arms loosely in lap and erect spine.

PRACTITIONER: *You may notice that your breath is cool when you breathe in through your nostrils, but warmer when you breathe out through your nostrils. Good. Now take a deep breath in through your nose, but this next breath out, breathe out through your mouth. Good, deep breath in through your nose to the count of 4, and out through your mouth to the count of 8.*

Model for the youth another minute of deep breathing, with feet flat on the floor, arms loosely in lap and erect spine.

PRACTITIONER: *Good. Let's take in one more deep breath in and out. Slowly we will open our eyes and return our awareness back into the room.*

Repeatedly engaging in this form of breathwork will help the youth become more focused, more aware of thoughts, and more relaxed. They can then begin to work toward other forms of mindfulness, including open awareness meditation (explored next). Note in this script the practitioner tells the youth that they can either close their eyes or soften their gaze. This is important as some youth, particularly those who have experienced trauma, may not be comfortable with, or could be activated by, closing their eyes completely. We recommend giving them the option to lower their gaze in a non-focused manner.

Open Awareness Meditation
Ages: 7 and older
Time: Varies

Open awareness meditation is one of the core skills in becoming more mindful of one's internal and external worlds (Jennings, 2015). As opposed to focused meditation, open awareness allows a youth to focus their observations on their surroundings through non-judgmental awareness and without getting caught up in their thoughts. Following is a description of various open awareness meditative practices that you can use when working with youth. It is important to explain to youth that mindfulness and meditative practices do not require them to be without thoughts. Having thoughts is completely normal. The goal of mindfulness and meditation is to change our relationship with our thoughts. We want to become more aware of our thoughts, just as we become more aware of the present moment. As Tolle (1999) describes it, mindfulness involves being aware when your mind has wandered from the present moment, recognizing it, and consciously bringing attention back to the present.

Five Senses Meditation. Initially, open awareness meditation can be challenging for adults and youth alike, particularly younger children. A five senses meditation may help a student in the beginning stages of a meditation practice. This practice can bring greater focus and awareness of our surroundings via the five senses: hearing, tasting, smelling, touching, and seeing. The goal of this meditation is to ground the youth in the present moment, and to begin to be aware of thoughts without attaching to or being absorbed by them. This practice can be used with children as young as preschool, with modified language for their development level. Again, it is best if the practitioner also does the exercise along with the youth.

When engaging youth in this meditation, begin by asking them to tell you what the five senses are. Name any that the youth leaves out. Then explain how we can use our five senses to help us pay better attention to what is going on around us.

PRACTITIONER: *One way to know what is happening around us is to use our five senses. We will take in several 4x8 breaths then close our eyes or soften our gaze and look down at the floor. As you continue with 4x8 breaths, listen to the sounds you can hear. Note some of these sounds. Next, notice the weight of your body in your chair, how your feet feel on the floor, the temperature of the air on your face and hands. Next, notice any taste on your tongue, and then any smells in the room. Now, open your eyes and look around the room. What do you see? Finally, take one last deep breath and exhale.*

Form 3.7 contains a complete Five Senses Script. Form 3.8 contains a variation of the Five Senses Script, using the youth's hand and five fingers as a tangible reminder for focusing on each of their senses in the present moment.

Specific Mindfulness Practices
Ages: 3 and older
Time: 5 minutes

Mindful Eating. Mindful eating can be a fun way to introduce and practice awareness of the present moment via the sense of taste. This technique uses the five senses to explore a food item, such as a raisin or piece of chocolate. Mindful eating has been embraced, not just in the mindfulness community as a technique for increasing awareness of the present moment, but also by practitioners who work with individuals with disordered eating behaviors (Atkinson & Wade, 2015). For example, mindfulness-based eating awareness can be used to successfully treat binge-eating disorder (Kristeller & Wolever, 2010). Eating food mindfully can lead to greater enjoyment of food and being satiated more quickly (Nelson, 2017).

A common way of practicing mindful eating with youth is to give them a piece of foil wrapped chocolate, such as a Hershey Kiss. Ask them to hold it in their hand and explain that they are going to pretend to be visitors from another planet and have never seen this new food before. Tell them we will use all five of our senses to investigate this object. Next, have them look at the object. What does it look like? What is the color and texture? What does the weight of it feel like in their hand? Hold the object to their ear as they slowly unwrap the object. Are there any sounds from it? Next, smell the object; breathe deeply as they hold it under their nose. Ask them to place the object on their tongue and just hold it there. What does it feel like? Can they taste anything? Now, have them slowly chew the object starting with just one bite. Does the object change as they bite it? Is there more flavor now? Pause as the youth chews the object. Now, tell them to swallow the object. Did they notice any taste left on their tongue? Finally ask how this was different from how they usually eat a piece of candy.

A script is provided for a mindful eating exercise in Form 3.9. After the exercise, give time for the youth to describe the experience. Note that though a piece of chocolate is used in this example, any bite-sized food item can be utilized (e.g., raisins).

Mindful Walking. Mindful walking is another activity that brings a present-focused manner to an ordinary, everyday experience. You will need some space to move around when introducing this activity. Being outdoors can help, if that is an option, (e.g., the fresh air, the crunching of leaves under foot).

You can introduce this technique by simply saying, "*Today we are going to be doing some mindful walking. As we walk, pay attention to how your weight shifts from the heel to the ball of the foot and the weight of your feet as they hit the ground.*" Demonstrate for the youth slow, mindful walking, overexaggerating each step. Model deep breathing during this exercise, when possible.

Mindful walking can also be incorporated into the Five Senses Script or Take Five activity (Form 3.7 and 3.8) by attending to the various senses during a walk. For example, instruct the youth to attend to the smell of the air, the temperature on their face and hands, and the sounds in the environment while walking. This form of mindfulness practice can be particularly helpful to use with children who are more active, have attentional concerns, or with younger children, wherein the practice needs to be more concrete, activity based, and tangible.

Gratitude and Heartfulness
Ages: 3 and older with adaptations
Time: Varies

Integrating gratitude and heartfulness work into a youth's mindfulness practice can improve social and emotional well-being. Emmons and McCullough (2003) found that a daily practice of listing things we are grateful for can improve mood. That which we focus on expands (Tolle, 1999). When we shift the spotlight of attention onto aspects of our lives that are healing, grounding, and healthy, this awareness can expand and positively affect our mental well-being. Hanson and Mendius (2009) call this process "taking in the good"; focusing on the things in life that we value and attending consciously to those things to internalize them. Research supports the use of gratitude journaling as a method for increasing youth's social well-being and engagement in the classroom (Flinchbaugh et al., 2012; Froh et al., 2010). Gratitude journaling can be as simple as giving the youth a notebook to record three things they are grateful for a couple of times each week. To help the youth establish gratitude as a routine, you can recommend that they write this list at bedtime and review it the following morning, thereby starting their day in a positive way. This type of nighttime gratitude journaling has been found to increase participant well-being across multiple outcome measures (Emmons and McCullough, 2003). A gratitude list can also be incorporated into a focused meditation. For example, as the youth is doing their 4x8 breathwork, they could focus mentally on one item from their gratitude list like a mantra (see Focused Attention Meditation section). A gratitude practice could be incorporated into work with almost any aged youth as long as they are cognitively able to construct such a list.

Heartfulness can be defined as the desire to bond and connect with others and the world (Daugherty, 2014). The Mindful Schools program (Mindful Schools, 2015a) defines heartfulness as having a warm, heartfelt relationship with whatever is happening in one's experience, internal or external, and developing the capacity to regard oneself, others, and the world with a sense of empathy and kindness. Research has supported linking the practices of mindfulness and heartfulness, with positive emotions as a mechanism of change in mindful practice. Integrating heartfulness has been used in research as an intervention strategy for assisting the cultivation of positive emotions (Fredrickson et al., 2008). Deliberate cultivation of compassion offers a new coping strategy that fosters positive affect, even when confronted with distressing stimuli (Klimecki et al., 2014). Heartfulness can be used across age levels, with variations as discussed next.

One heartful strategy involves offering a kind wish to oneself or someone else while doing deep, mindful breathing. Wishing someone peace, calm, or health can be a positive heartful meditation during breathwork for elementary aged youth to adulthood (Mindful Schools, 2015a). The practitioner can tell the youth to imagine the person in their mind as they silently repeat to themselves, "I wish you peace. I wish you calm. I wish you health." This activity can be combined with deep breathing techniques.

For younger children, a more concrete activity can be offered. Gordon and Borushok (2019) suggest a heartful strategy wherein the practitioner asks the youth to imagine that an inanimate object, such as a stuffed animal, is in a difficult situation. First, instruct the youth to give that animal comfort and compassion such as holding the animal and saying reassuring, kind words. Then, encourage the youth to extend that compassion toward themselves. This concrete strategy can be used with children as young as preschool-age.

Yoga
Ages: 3 and older with adaptations
Time: Varies

Yoga consists of coordinating breathwork, meditation, and specific postures to focus and calm the mind (Feuerstein, 2003). Yoga has been found to be an effective intervention in helping to reduce anxiety and aggression and increase mental well-being in youth (Hagen & Nayar, 2014; Stueck & Gloeckner, 2005). Research using yoga with pediatric populations suggests that yoga can be an effective intervention to improve physical functioning, cardiorespiratory health, and behavior in children and adolescents, though more studies are recommended (Galantino et al., 2008).

Based on a child's developmental age, physical fitness, and setting of practice, you can adapt the length and type of practice, along with the challenge of poses. Cultural considerations as it relates to yoga practice is more fully explored in Chapter 7.

When beginning any yoga practice, start in a relaxed pose, such as a seated, cross-legged position, to allow for initial breathwork. Any of the breathwork practices overviewed earlier in this chapter are an appropriate beginning to a yoga session. The physical environment should be spacious enough to give everyone room to move during their practice without bumping into a desk, object, or another person. Shoes are typically not worn, and ideally a non-slip mat is available for use. Tell the youth that yoga should not hurt or cause pain in their body. If they notice pain, they should loosen their pose or stop the pose altogether. Form 3.10 contains some basic yoga poses for beginning yoga instruction with youth.

When conducting yoga with younger children, the use of metaphors can be helpful in demonstrating different poses. For example, animals and objects are often used in posture instruction, such as cat, cow, or tree pose (see Form 3.10; White, 2009). The idea is both to assist in the child's form through the use of these metaphors, but also to make the practice fun so that they will remain engaged and continue the practice.

When wrapping up the yoga practice, a transition period of rest is often helpful to quiet the body and mind. This may include lying down, with eyes closed, on the floor in a supine position (relaxation pose) and focusing on the breath, a sound such as music, a repetitive phrase, or a visualization exercise (White, 2009). The suggestion can be made to the youth that the relaxed, peaceful, and calm feelings in their body and mind will remain with them into the rest of their day.

The Use of Technology for Individual Practice

Computer and phone applications can encourage students to practice mindfulness outside of the school setting. Some apps, such as Headspace Inc. (2022) and Wellbeyond Meditation for Kids (2020) provide breathing exercises, visualizations, and various meditations. Other apps can assist youth in their yoga practice, such as Super Stretch Yoga (2017), which offers yoga poses with animations, video, and instruction using

Table 3.3 Mindfulness apps for youth.

Name	Target Age	Description
Chill (2020)	4+	Encourages daily mindfulness practice by sending up to five random reminders to mediate, as well as serene quotes and photos that can be shared via social media.
Dreamykid Meditation (2020)	3–17	Offers general and issue-based meditations, guided visualizations, and affirmations that are updated monthly, as well as ambient background noise, strategies for focus and more.
Headspace Inc. (2022)	>5–12	Provides breathing exercises, visualizations, and themed focus-based meditations, including calm, focus, kindness, sleep, and wake-up. Meditations are tailored for separate age groups.
Smiling Mind (2022)	7+	Offers youth-tailored meditation programs, reminders, and a dashboard for tracking mindful progress.
Stop, Breathe & Think (2022)	5–10	Provides youth-oriented mindfulness games in which youth can check into how they are feeling using emojis and participate in mindful activities tied to those emotions. Youth are rewarded with stickers as they make progress.
Super Stretch Yoga (2017)	4+	Offers 12 yoga poses with animations, video, and instruction using animated characters.
Wellbeyond Meditation for Kids (2020)	6–13	Offers five meditations, including sleep, kindness, feelings, focus, and centering that range from 3 to 14 minutes in length. Uses child friendly images and tones throughout the app.

animated characters. Practitioners, after familiarizing themselves with the available technology, can consider suggesting certain apps that could be helpful for youth to continue their mindfulness practice at home or on the go.

Table 3.3 lists a variety of applications that can be downloaded on a computer or smart-phone device. Some are free, whereas others are available for a small fee. This list is not exhaustive, and technology is ever changing, so practitioners are encouraged to explore various apps for themselves first in order to find what may be the best match for their students.

Case Examples

The following are two case examples illustrating mindfulness practices with two youth of different ages.

Colette, Age 5
Presenting Concern: Anxiety and Somatic Complaints

Colette (she/her/hers), a kindergartener, is referred for individual counseling services because she is having anxiety symptoms in her classroom, often stomachaches and headaches. Before meeting with Colette, the practitioner gathered background information and symptom presentation from Colette's mother and her teacher. Colette often appears visibly anxious, fidgeting and, at times, crying in the classroom when she feels overwhelmed or stressed. The practitioner decided to use mindfulness to help Colette reduce her anxiety and somatic symptoms.

In session 1, the practitioner began her work with Colette by sharing with her in simple terms how stress affects the body, using the following analogy: If a bear were to enter the room, we would likely hold our breath or take short, quick breaths. This would make our bodies ready to run really fast or fight the bear. But if this fear and tension goes on for a long time, it can make our bodies feel tired and even sick, giving us upset stomachs and headaches. This led into a short conversation about how the things we think to ourselves can act like "bears," making us feel scared or worried, even if there isn't an actual bear in the room.

In this initial session, the practitioner also taught Colette how to use 3x6 breaths (an age adaptation of 4x8 breaths). Colette laid down in the relaxation pose (Form 3.2) and watched as a small stuffed animal rose and fell with her diaphragmatic breaths. This technique was chosen to help Colette decrease her SNS arousal and to help set the stage for further mindfulness work. To help Colette better understand the practice, she was also told to imagine breathing in the scent of flowers and blowing out birthday candles. Bubbles were also given to Colette as a playful way to remember to practice her deep in breath and elongated outbreath. The practitioner encouraged her to use her 3x6 breaths daily over the next week, and also contacted her teacher and mother to help remind Colette to practice. The practitioner also briefly taught Colette's teacher and mother how to use 3x6 breathing, so that they could model this strategy for Colette at home and in the classroom.

In session two, the practitioner used the body scan script (Form 3.6) to help Colette become aware of tension in her body, as she had numerous somatic complaints associated with her anxiety, and to couple the body scan with the 3x6 breaths. Colette responded very well to the script. The practitioner gave her mother a copy of the script to begin to practice these skills at home each night before bedtime.

In sessions three and four, mindful eating with a piece of foil wrapped chocolate (Form 3.9) and mindful walking were added into Colette's practice after modeling by the practitioner. These activities helped make her mindfulness practice more tangible. In session five, the simple yoga poses included in Form 3.10 were practiced with Colette to further assist with the mind-body connection. A copy of these poses was given to Colette's mother for follow up practice at home. In sessions six through eight, focused meditation was used with Colette. It coupled her 3x6 breathing with a repeated mantra of "I am safe. I am calm." The practitioner met with her for two additional sessions, for a total of ten sessions, to continue practicing and refining all mindfulness strategies learned over the course of treatment.

At six-week follow up, both parent and teacher report noted a significant improvement in Colette's anxious behavior and somatic complaints.

Jack, Age 14
Presenting Concern: Attentional Issues and Depression

Jack (he/him/his) is a freshman in high school. He was referred by his mother and math teacher for challenges with focus and also some depressive symptoms, such as negative self-talk, withdrawn behavior, and a lack of motivation. Jack presented as somewhat sullen in the first session with the practitioner. He noted that he has long struggled in school and that he had been previously diagnosed with ADHD in elementary school, at which point he was prescribed a stimulant medication to help with focus. He said he often becomes distracted by his daydreams and so it is challenging to follow instructions in the classroom. With Jack doubting his academic abilities, particularly in math, it was clear to the practitioner that these challenges had begun to hurt Jack's self-esteem. Jack mentioned to the practitioner that he frequently tells himself, "I can't do it." and "Why even try?" The practitioner decided to use mindfulness interventions with Jack.

In the first session, the practitioner started with psychoeducation explaining how thoughts can be incredibly distracting and also distorted and hurtful (see section Educating Youth on Stress, Their Bodies, and Mindfulness of this chapter). This helped Jack to understand that, though his thoughts are troublesome, they are also common. The practitioner asked Jack if he ever loses things or forgets to do things. Jack acknowledged this happens quite a bit. The practitioner then discussed how, when we get really distracted by our thinking minds, it takes us out of the present moment, making it more likely that we will lose track of things around us. A basic overview of mindfulness, along with the benefits of the practice, was then given to Jack to aid with buy-in.

In session two, the practitioner worked with Jack on beginning 4x8 breaths in seated posture (Form 3.3). Jack took well to this technique and agreed to begin using it in between sessions. The practitioner built upon this in session three, using a focused awareness meditation with Jack, with breath being the object of focus. The practitioner explained that Jack's breath is like an anchor. When thoughts pull him "out to sea," he can use his breath to anchor him back to the present moment.

These techniques were selected to decrease Jack's negative, ruminative thoughts and help him increase a sense of physical and mental calmness.

In sessions three and four, the practitioner introduced the Five Senses Script (Form 3.7), as well as the Take Five (Form 3.8) activity, and encouraged him to practice these skills each day in between sessions. These techniques made the mindfulness work more tangible for Jack, allowing him to practice the activities by himself outside of the sessions. The more practice Jack had with the techniques, the more progress he began to experience.

Jack noted for the practitioner that he was beginning to become more aware of his surroundings through the use of the mindfulness skills. He had increased focus in the classroom by coming back into the present moment to refocus on the lectures. In session five, the practitioner suggested Jack begin a gratitude journal to foster positive thinking.

In the sixth and final session with Jack, the apps Headspace and Chill were recommended to aid with ongoing practice of the mindfulness strategies discussed over the course of treatment. Jack downloaded them onto his phone during the session. (See the section on the Use of Technology). Jack had become more focused, had healthier cognitions about himself, and felt empowered that he could control his attention beyond just taking his medication every morning. Jack's mother and math teacher also both reported improvement in Jack's mood and attention.

Conclusion

Mindfulness practices cover a wide array of techniques, including breathwork, meditation, the mindful use of senses, and yoga. This chapter presented a select group of techniques well suited for individual use with youth in the school setting. By no means is this chapter a comprehensive review of mindfulness practices. However, with the variety of tools offered here, mindfulness can be a powerful and portable skill for youth. In fact, mindfulness meditation made news when 12 Thai children were trapped in a cave for several weeks. Their soccer coach, Ekapol Chanthawong, had led the boys on the hike and had been trained in meditation before becoming a soccer coach. Over their two-week ordeal, he taught the boys the techniques to help keep them calm. It is thought that the meditation practices in the cave allowed them to preserve their energy and survive (Barclay, 2018). As the great Buddhist Zen Master, Hanh (2012), eloquently wrote,

> When we practice mindfulness, we can take our practice with us wherever we go, just like you take your phone with you; but mindfulness doesn't take up any space or make your bag any heavier, and your batteries never run down. Whenever you go somewhere, your practice goes with you.
>
> (pg. 77)

Form 3.1

Diaphragmatic Breathing: Crocodile Pose
Materials Needed: Perhaps a thin pillow or blanket
Age Adaptations: None
Best Used For: Beginning diaphragmatic breathing exercises

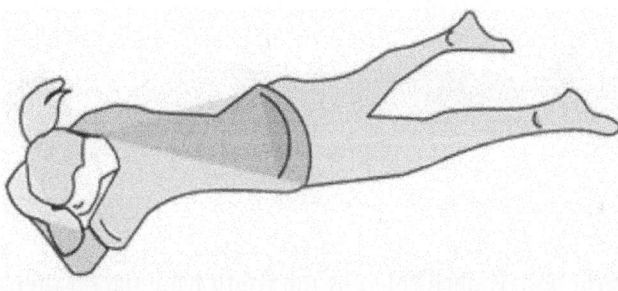

Crocodile pose is performed by lying comfortably on the floor face down. The youth may rest their forehead on their folded forearms, elevating the upper chest slightly off of the floor. If that is uncomfortable for them, they may prop their upper body with a thin pillow or a blanket (draping their chin over the prop).

Form 3.2

> **Diaphragmatic Breathing: Relaxation Pose**
> **Materials Needed**: Perhaps a thin pillow or blanket
> **Age Adaptations**: None
> **Best Used For**: Diaphragmatic breathing exercises or a meditative exercise

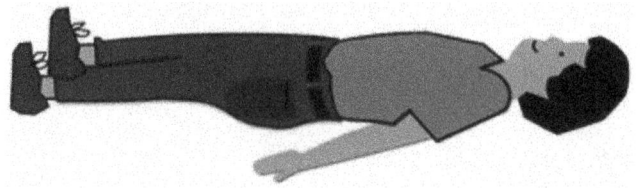

Relaxation pose is performed by the youth lying flat on their back on a flat surface. A yoga mat or blanket can be used. Their head and neck can be supported with a thin pillow or blanket, if desired. Arms and legs should rest comfortably off to the side.

Form 3.3

> **Diaphragmatic Breathing: Seated Posture**
> **Materials Needed**: A chair
> **Age Adaptations**: None
> **Best Used For**: Diaphragmatic breathing exercises or a meditative exercise

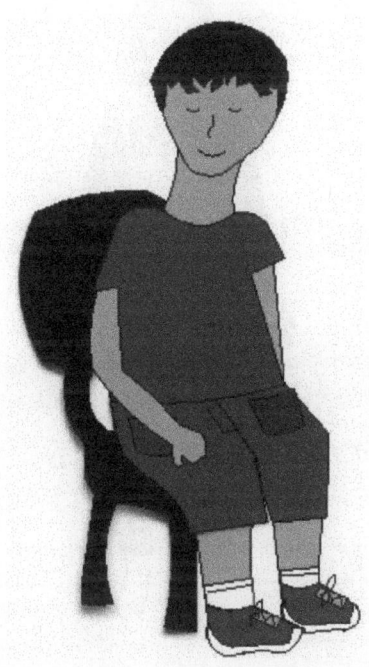

In seated posture, the youth will sit erect in any seated pose, such as sitting on a flat seated chair. The youth will loosely rest their hands in their laps, with straight spine and softened gaze or eyes closed.

Form 3.4

Diaphragmatic Breathing: Mountain Pose
Materials Needed: None
Age Adaptations: None
Best Used For: Diaphragmatic breathing exercises or yoga poses

---

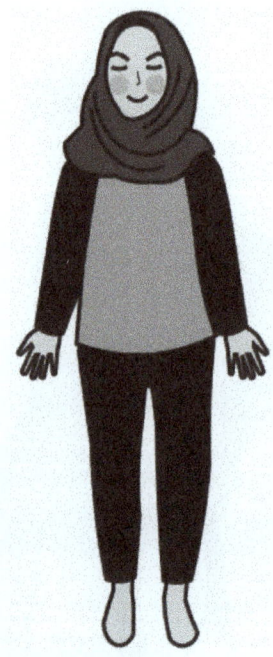

Mountain Pose, or Tadasana, is where the youth will stand with feet flat on the floor, slightly apart. Spine should be erect, and arms should be hung beside the torso, palms slightly out.

Form 3.5

Alternate Nostril Breathing (ANB)
Materials Needed: None
Age Adaptations: Ages 10 and older
Best Used For: Youth who are experiencing anxiety symptoms

Begin by having the youth sit in a quiet posture, such as seated posture as displayed in Form 3.3 or sitting crossed legged on the floor. Have the youth bring their right hand up to the nose and fold the index and the middle fingers so that the right thumb can be used to close the right nostril and the index finger can be used to close the left nostril.

Using the right thumb, have the youth softly close the right nostril, and inhale as slowly as they can through the left nostril, then closing it with their index finger. Pause briefly, then have them open and exhale

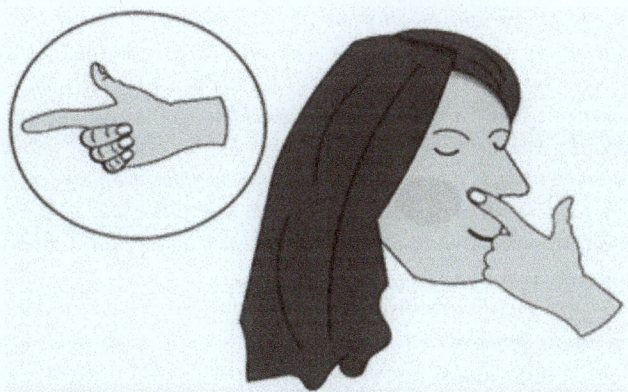

slowly through the right nostril. With the right nostril open, inhale slowly, then have them close it with their thumb. Pause briefly, then have them exhale through the left nostril. Once their exhalation is complete, have them inhale through the left. Pause before having them move to the right. Repeat this pattern five to ten times.

Form 3.6

Body Scan Script
Materials Needed: Perhaps a thin pillow or blanket
Age Adaptations: This script can be used with preschool aged children on up, with some adjustment of language.
Best Used For: Youth experiencing anxiety, stress, or somatic complaints

Begin with breathing exercises.

Today, we are going to do a quick body scan. This involves focusing our attention on any sensations we might be having in our bodies. We aren't trying to change these sensations, just notice them.

Breath: *First, let's turn our attention to our breath. Continue taking some 4x8 breaths. As you do, see if you can notice what the air feels like as you first breathe in. Is the air cold or warm as it enters your mouth/nose? See if you can follow your breath from the moment it enters your mouth/nose, until it enters your lungs. Notice how your body feels different as the air enters your lungs. Finally, follow your breath as it exits your body. Has the temperature of the air changed? Does your body feel any different?*

Feet: *Next, I want you to turn your attention to your feet. See if you can notice how your feet feel as they make contact with the floor. Do your feet feel warm or cold, tense or relaxed? Take a moment to just notice your feet. And if your attention starts to drift to other thoughts, just notice that, and bring your attention back to your feet.*

Legs: *Now let's focus our attention on our legs. See if you can notice how it feels for your pants to make contact with your legs. Are your legs feeling calm or do they want to move? Are they feeling heavy or light? Just take a moment to notice any sensations in your legs.*

Stomach: *Okay, now let's pay attention to our tummies. Notice how your tummy changes as you breathe in and out. See if you can identify any other sensations your tummy might be feeling. Are you full or hungry? Can you feel your shirt making contact with your tummy? Spend a few moments to just notice any sensations happening in your tummy. And if you notice that your mind has wandered off, gently bring your focus back to your tummy.*

Hands: *Good, now we are going to shift our focus to our hands. Notice where your hands are currently located. Are they in your lap, holding onto the chair, or clasped together? Are they feeling cold or warm; tense or relaxed? No need to move them or do anything with them. Just take a moment to notice them.*

Arms: *Next, we are going to pay attention to our arms. How are your arms positioned? Try tuning your attention into noticing what your arms are* *coming into contact with. Are your arms feeling heavy or light? Do you notice any tingling, goosebumps, or other sensations?*

Chest: *Now, shift your focus to your chest. See if you can focus your mind on simply following the rise and fall of your chest as you continue to breathe in and out. Follow this rise and fall for several breaths. If you notice your mind has been wandering, simply bring your attention back to noticing the rise and fall of your chest.*

Shoulders: *Let's pay attention to our shoulders now. Notice the positioning of your shoulders. Are they tense or loose; are they raised or relaxed? Spend a few moments just focused on noticing any sensations in your shoulders.*

Face: *Finally, center your focus on your face and head. What type of expression do you have on your face right now? As you are tuning in your focus, notice if you feel any desire to change your facial expression. If your facial expression has changed since paying attention to your facial muscles, notice any changes to the sensations you are experiencing.*

End by taking a few final 4x8 breaths.

Form 3.7

Five Senses Script.
Age Adaptations: None
Best Used For: Giving youth tangible guidance for how to combine present moment awareness with breathwork. Good for any presenting concern.

Now we are going to use our five senses to help us to be right here in this moment. Can you tell me what the five senses are? Seeing is one.

Wait for response, filling in the others (hearing, tasting, touching, smelling) if missed by the child.

That's right, those are all of our senses. Using all of our five senses can help us pay better attention to what is going on around us and help our bodies calm down!

We will start by taking in a few deep breaths, as we have been working on. A deep breath in through our nose to the count of 4, hold it briefly, then out to the count of 8. Good, let's do another.

Model with the youth taking in these deep breaths. Take four deep breaths with them.

Good, now, either soften your eyes, without focusing hard on any one thing, and look towards the floor or, if you are comfortable with it, close your eyes.

Model this for the youth.

As we continue to take in those deep 4 by 8 breaths, we will turn our attention to just what we are hearing right now in the room.

Here note for the youth what sounds are being heard either in or outside the room. The following sample can be modified as to what is being heard in that moment.

Perhaps you hear the sound of the air conditioner, or the clock ticking. You may hear sounds outside the room, like people talking or traffic going by. Just focus on your deep breaths, and what you are hearing right now.

Good, now notice the weight of your body in your chair. Notice the solidness of the floor underneath your feet. Note the temperature of the air on your face and hands. We will continue to take our deep breaths in to the count of 4, and out to the count of 8.

Notice if you have any taste on your tongue. Note if you can smell any smells or scents in the room.

Now open your eyes and look around the room. You may notice that colors seem brighter, and lines on objects are sharper and clearer. Perhaps you notice something in the room that you had not noticed before.

Good, and we will take in one last deep breath, and let it out.

Be sure to ask the youth how that was for them and have them describe what it was like to use their five senses in this way.

Form 3.8

Take Five

Age Adaptations: None

Best Used For: A variation on the Five Senses activity, giving youth tangible guidance for how to combine present moment awareness with breathwork. Good for any presenting concern.

Instruct the youth to use their fingers to remind them of a tangible way to practice mindful awareness. Note: you can photocopy the following and give it to the youth to remind them of the practice.

- -

TAKE 5! Right Now:

Table 3.4

5	Name 5 things you can see
4	Name 4 things you can touch
3	Name 3 things you can hear
2	Name 2 things you can smell
1	Name 1 thing you can taste

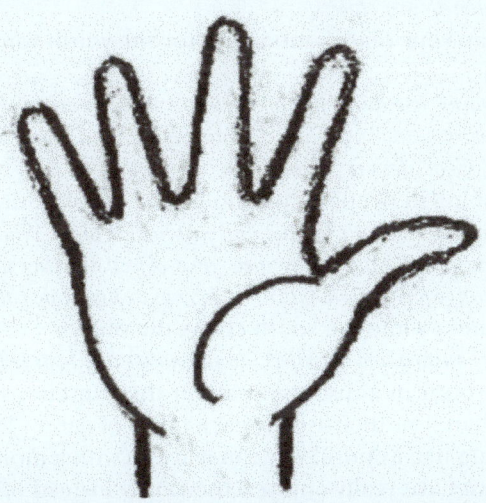

> **Form 3.9**
>
> **Mindful Eating Exercise**
> **Age Adaptations:** None
> **Best Used For:** Giving youth tangible guidance for how to combine present moment awareness with breathwork. Good for any presenting concern.

Give the youth a piece of foil wrapped chocolate, such as a Hershey's Kiss. Tell them not to eat the chocolate, but instead to hold the chocolate in their hand.

Script:

> *While holding the chocolate in your hand, we are going to pretend like we are visitors from another planet and are experiencing this new food for the first time. We are going to use all of our five senses to investigate this object.*

Model holding the chocolate between your index finger and thumb, bringing it up to your face.

Look at the object as you hold it in your fingers. Notice what it looks like. Is it shiny or dull, bumpy or smooth? What color is it? Does the light catch the object on some areas differently than others? What does the weight of the chocolate feel like in your hand?

Next, we are going to use our sense of hearing to listen to hear if we hear any sounds as we unwrap our objects.

Slowly unwrap your object, modeling for the youth your intense focus on the process.

Now we are going use our sense of smell to smell the object. Breathe deeply as you hold your object under your nose. Notice if you can smell any scents as you breath in deeply. Good, let's try that again.

Model breathing in deeply as you hold the chocolate under your nose.

Now, place the object on your tongue and just hold it there. What does it feel like? Can you taste anything? Now slowly chew your object, starting with just one bite. Does the object change form as you bite it? Is there more flavor now that you can taste?

Pause a moment while the youth chews the object.

Good, now, as you swallow the object, do you notice any taste left on your tongue?

Engage the youth in a discussion about the exercise, asking how this was different than how they usually eat a piece of candy. Discuss with the youth that eating in a mindful way can leave us with a more satisfied feeling after, like we have really enjoyed the candy instead of quickly eating it without having awareness of it.

Form 3.10

A Sampling of Basic Yoga Poses
Cat

Cow

Tree

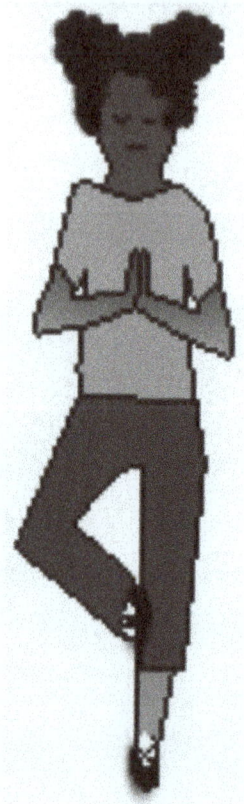

Child's

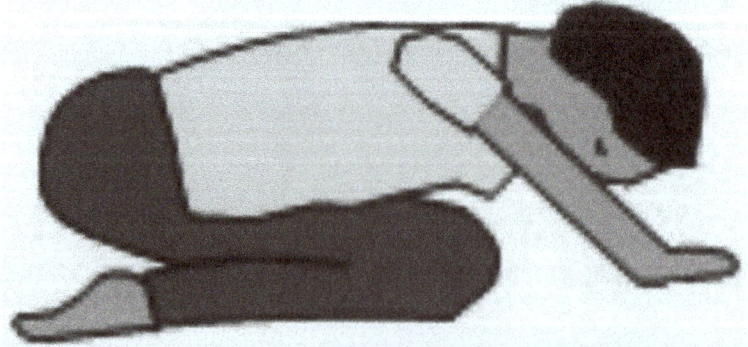

Downward Dog

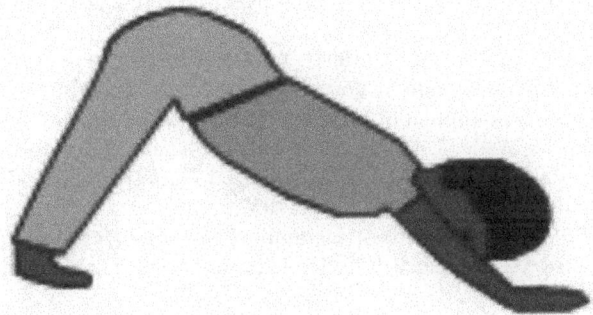

Mountain

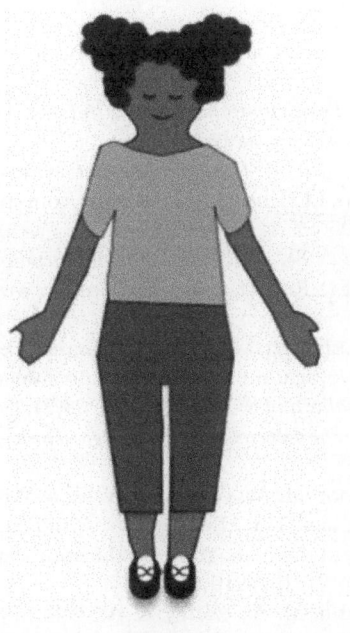

Relaxation

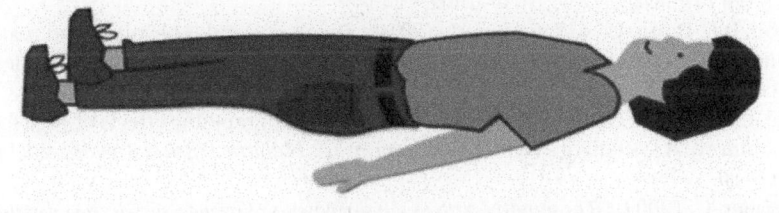

References

Adhana, R., Gupta, R., Dvivedi, J., & Ahmad, S. (2013). The influence of the 2:1 yogic breathing technique on essential hypertension. *Indian Journal of Physiological Pharmacology, 57*(1), 38–44.

Asmundson, G. J., & Stein, M. B. (1994). Vagal attenuation in panic disorder: An assessment of parasympathetic nervous system function and subjective reactivity to respiratory manipulations. *Psychosomatic Medicine, 56*(3), 187–193.

Atkinson, M. J., & Wade, T. D. (2015). Mindfulness-based prevention for eating disorders: A school-based cluster randomized controlled study. *International Journal of Eating Disorders, 48*(7), 1024–1037.

Barclay, E. (2018). How Buddhist meditation kept the Thai boys calm in the cave. *Vox.* www.vox.com/2018/7/9/17548512/thai-cave-rescue-soccer-boys-meditation-buddhism

Chill. (2020). *Chill – mindfulness reminders* (Version 1.5.16) [Mobile app]. Minima Software, LLC. https://apps.apple.com/us/app/chill-mindfulness-reminders/id986509491

Clark, J. (2019). *Soothe your nervous system with 2–1 breathing.* Yoga International. https://yogainternational.com/article/view/soothe-your-nervous-system-with-2-to-1-breathing

Daugherty, A. (2014). *From mindfulness to heartfulness: A journey of transformation through the science of embodiment.* Balboa Press.

Dreamykid Meditation. (2020). *Dreamykid meditation* (Version 1.6) [Mobile app]. Chiron Media Group, LLC. https://apps.apple.com/us/app/dreamykid-meditation-app/id1430696683

Elliott, S. (2010, January 8). *Diaphragm mediates action of autonomic and enteric nervous systems.* BMED Report: Psychophysiology. www.bmedreport.com/archives/8309.

Emmons, R. A., & McCullough, M. E. (2003). Counting blessings versus burdens: An experimental investigation of gratitude and subjective well-being in daily life. *Journal of Personality and Social Psychology, 84*(2), 377–389.

Feuerstein, G. (2003). *The deeper dimension of yoga: Theory and practice.* Shambhala Publications.

Flinchbaugh, C. L., Moore, E. W. G., Chang, Y. K., & May, D. R. (2012). Student well-being interventions: The effects of stress management techniques and gratitude journaling in the management education classroom. *Journal of Management Education, 36*(2), 191–219.

Fredrickson, B. L., Cohn, M. A., Coffey, K. A., Pek, J., & Finkel, S. M. (2008). Open hearts build lives: Positive emotions, induced through loving-kindness meditation, build consequential personal resources. *Journal of Personality and Social Psychology, 95*(5), 1045–1062.

Froh, J. J., Bono, G., & Emmons, R. (2010). Being grateful is beyond good manners: Gratitude and motivation to contribute to society among early adolescents. *Motivation and Emotion, 34*(2), 144–157.

Galantino, M. L., Galbavy, R., & Quinn, L. (2008). Therapeutic effects of yoga for children: A systematic review of the literature. *Pediatric Physical Therapy, 20*(1), 66–80.

Germer, C. (2009). *The mindful path to self-compassion: Freeing yourself from destructive thoughts and emotions.* Guilford Press.

Gordon, T., & Borushok, J. (2019). *Acceptance and mindfulness toolbox for children and adolescents.* PESI Publishing and Media.

Hagen, I., & Nayar, U. S. (2014). Yoga for children and young people's mental health and well-being: Research review and reflections on the mental health potentials of yoga. *Frontiers in Psychiatry, 5,* 35.

Hanh, T. N. (2012). *Fear: Essential wisdom for getting through the storm.* Random House.

Hanson, R., & Mendius, R. (2009). *Buddha's brain: The practical neuroscience of happiness, love, and wisdom.* New Harbinger Publication.

Headspace Inc. (2022). *Headspace* (Version 3.209.0) [Mobile app]. Mac app store. https://apps.apple.com/us/app/headspace-mindful-meditation/id4931 45008

Jennings, P. A. (2015). *Mindfulness for teachers: Simple skills for peace and productivity in the classroom (the Norton series on the social neuroscience of education).* W.W. Norton & Company.

Kabat-Zinn, J. (2003). Mindfulness-based interventions in context: Past, present, and future. *Clinical Psychology: Science and Practice, 10*(2), 144–156.

Klimecki, O. M., Leiberg, S., Ricard, M., & Singer, T. (2014). Differential pattern of functional brain plasticity after compassion and empathy training. *Social Cognitive and Affective Neuroscience, 9*(6), 873–879.

Kristeller, J. L., & Wolever, R. Q. (2010). Mindfulness-based eating awareness training for treating binge eating disorder: The conceptual foundation. *Eating Disorders, 19*(1), 49–61.

Mindful Schools. (2015a). *Mindfulness fundamentals.* www.mindfulschools.org/training/mindfulness-fundamentals/

Nelson, J. B. (2017). Mindful eating: The art of presence while you eat. *Diabetes Spectrum: A Publication of the American Diabetes Association, 30*(3), 171–174.

Nestor, J. (2020). *Breath: The new science of a lost art.* Riverhead Books.

Oneda, B., Ortega, K. C., Gusmao, J. L., Araujo, T. G., & Mion, D. (2010). Sympathetic nerve activity is decreased during device-guided slow breathing. *Hypertension Research, 33*(7), 708–712.

Rechtschaffen, D. (2016). *The mindful education workbook: Lessons for teaching mindfulness to students.* W.W. Norton & Company.

Renshaw, T. L., & Cook, C. R. (2017). Introduction to the special issue: Mindfulness in the schools – historical roots, current status, and future directions. *Psychology in the Schools, 54,* 5–12.

Seppala, E., Bradley, C., & Goldstein, M. R. (2020). Research: Why breathing is so effective at reducing stress. *Harvard Business Review.* https://store.hbr.org/product/research-why-breathing-is-so-effective-at-reducing-stress/h05vns?sku=H05VNS-PDF-ENG

Sinha, A., Deepak, D., & Gusain, V. (2013). Assessment of the effects of pranayama/alternate nostril breathing on the parasympathetic nervous system in young adults. *Journal of Clinical and Diagnostic Research, 7*(5), 821–823.

Smiling Mind. (2022). *Smiling mind: Meditation for all ages* (Version 4.10.0) [Mobile app]. Mac App Store. https://apps.apple.com/us/app/smiling-mind/id560 442518

Smith, S. T. (2011). *The user's guide to the human mind: Why our brains make us unhappy, anxious, and neurotic and what we can do about it.* New Harbinger Publications.

Stop, Breathe & Think. (2022). *Stop breathe think: Meditation* (Version 10.3) [Mobile app]. Mac App Store. https://apps.apple.com/us/app/stop-breathe-think-meditation/id778848692

Stueck, M., & Gloeckner, N. (2005). Yoga for children in the mirror of the science: Working spectrum and practice fields of the training of relaxation with elements of yoga for children. *Early Child Development and Care, 175*(4), 371–377.

Super Stretch Yoga. (2017). *Super Stretch Yoga* (Version 1.2.1) [Mobile app]. The Adventures of Super Stretch, LLC. https://apps.apple.com/us/app/super-stretch-yoga/id456113661

Telles, S., Sharma, S. K., & Balkrishna, A. (2014). Blood pressure and heart rate variability during yoga-based alternate nostril breathing practice and breath awareness. *Medical Science Monitor Basic Research, 20*, 184–193.

Tolle, E. (1999). *The power of now: A guide to spiritual enlightenment.* New World Library.

Walker, J., & Pacik, D. (2017). Controlled rhythmic yogic breathing as complementary treatment for post-traumatic stress disorder in military veterans: A case series. *Medical Acupuncture, 29*(3), 232–238.

Wellbeyond Meditation for Kids. (2020). *Wellbeyond meditation for kids – kids mindfulness meditation* (Version 2.2) [Mobile app]. Wellbeyond, Inc. https://apps.apple.com/us/app/wellbeyond/id1082891966

White, L. (2009). Yoga for children. *Pediatric Nursing, 35*(5), 277–283, 295.

Zelano, C., Jiang, H., Zhou, G., Arora, N., Schuele, S., Rosenow, J., & Gottfried, J. A. (2016). Nasal respiration entrains human limbic oscillations and modulates cognitive function. *Journal of Neuroscience, 36*(49), 12448–12467.

Zelazo, P. D., & Lyons, K. E. (2012). Mindfulness training in childhood. *Human Development, 54*(2), 61–65.

4 ACT Strategies for Individual Work

Roadmap to Chapter 4

This chapter describes how to use ACT practices with mindfulness work.

- an overview of the ACT hexaflex model
- how to introduce attachment and acceptance of thoughts
- how to loosen attachments to thoughts and increase flexibility in thinking
- setting intentions and goals
- preparing the student for setbacks and relapse prevention

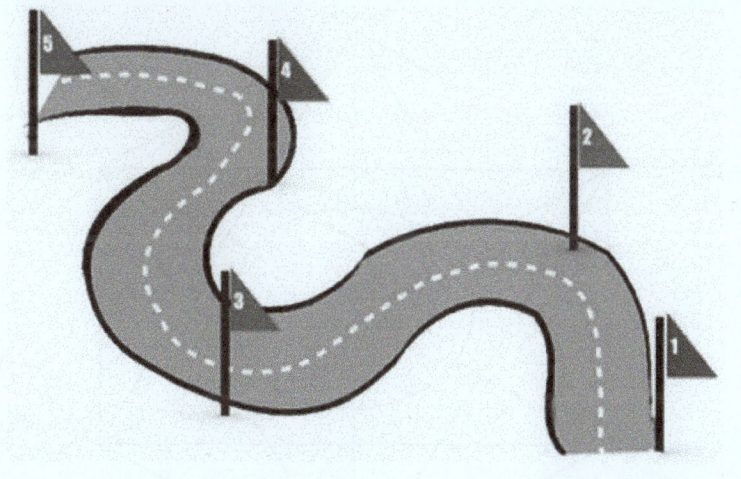

ACT is part of the "third wave" of behavioral therapies, incorporating mindfulness practice into cognitive and behavioral treatment (Hayes, 2004). Acceptance techniques can be used with almost any presenting concern. As discussed in Chapter 2, acceptance and commitment work

DOI: 10.4324/9781003318101-4

has been found to be effective with youth and adults experiencing both internalizing concerns, such as anxiety and depression, and externalizing concerns, such as anger management challenges. This chapter begins by explaining the ACT model in more detail and then presenting specific practices to use with students.

The Hexaflex Model in ACT

Six key areas are central to ACT: being present, acceptance, cognitive defusion, self-as-context, values, and committed action. (See Figure 4.1). Each contributes to the overall goal of increasing psychological flexibility. Psychological flexibility is the ability to be in the present moment, with full awareness, and openness to the experience, with goals and action guided by values. Each of these areas will be described next.

Attention to the Present Moment (Mindfulness)

Attention to the present moment simply means living flexibly in the here and now. Mindfulness is an awareness process, rather than a thinking process. Mindfulness involves being open to the present moment, even if the present moment involves discomfort and pain. The past is

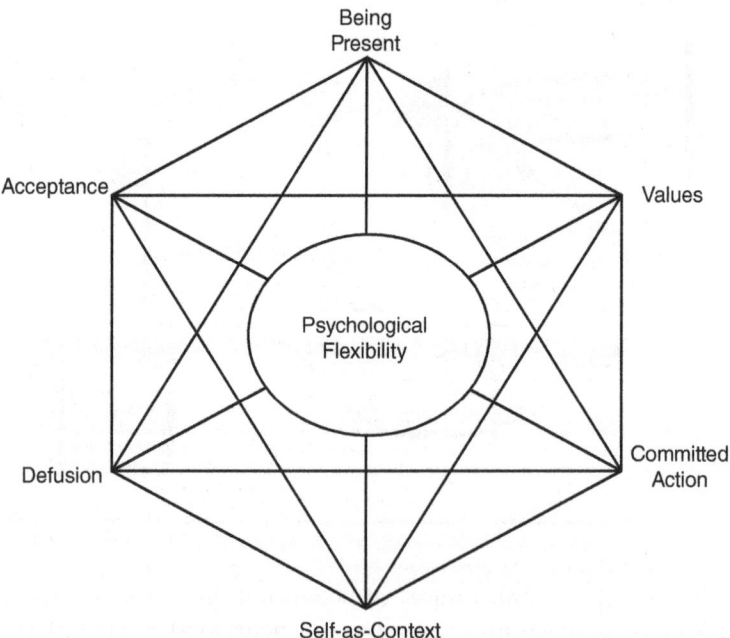

Figure 4.1 ACT's Hexaflex Model.

gone forever, and the future is yet to come. The past and the future are actually constructions made of stories and memories in our minds. These stories and memories can be so distracting that we miss what is going on around us. In the ACT framework, time is only a measure of change, and there is only the now in which to create that change (Hayes et al., 2012).

Acceptance

Experiential avoidance is the act of trying to block unpleasant thoughts and feelings. This avoidance can actually maintain and escalate the distress. Acceptance is an alternative to experiential avoidance. Acceptance, in ACT, is the adoption of an intentionally open, flexible, receptive, and nonjudgmental posture toward present-moment experience (Hayes et al., 2012). It is important to note that acceptance is not a giving up or giving in; instead, it is a willingness to turn toward things as they really are (Hayes, 2005). This can, in turn, allow for informed choice, as opposed to feeling mired in the resistance to reality.

Cognitive Defusion

Humans have the ability to translate experiences into words. Hayes (2005) calls this "the word machine." Our minds are continuously comparing, evaluating, predicting, and planning (Hayes et al., 2012). While words and language can be advantageous, they can also cause problems. They can facilitate negative thinking patterns and cause us to label ourselves, others, and the world in unhealthy or destructive ways. "Cognitive fusion" is the process of our thoughts dominating our experiences and behaviors (Harris, 2009). It's when we mistake thoughts for facts. Often, we get stuck in rule-bound living, fixating on the belief that there is only one right and true answer to any given question. This can become problematic to our mental health and flexibility in living. Cognitive defusion, on the other hand, is the ability to separate and create distance from thoughts (Harris, 2009). When we create distance from our thoughts, we can begin to recognize them for what they are – just thoughts, with no reality other than as mental events. With this recognition, we have more choices for how we respond and behave.

Self-as-Context

Self-as-context is essentially "awareness of our own awareness" (Harris, 2009). It is the observing mind or self that is aware that it is having thoughts (Hayes et al., 2012). When we say, "I notice my thoughts," the "I" is the observing self, or self-as-context. ACT describes three senses of self: the conceptualized self, self-as-awareness, and self-as-context. The conceptualized self is our self-description; this includes our thoughts, feelings, judgments, memories, and ideas about our identity. Self-as-awareness is the process of noticing and being in the present moment. Self-as-context is the part of the self "doing the noticing." In ACT, self-as-context can facilitate cognitive defusion and acceptance. Once we understand the concept of the observing self, we can better understand how to simply observe and accept thoughts and feelings (Harris, 2009; Hayes et al., 2012).

Values

In the ACT model, values are chosen life directions (Hayes, 2005). Values are distinct and separate from wants, needs, virtues, morals, ethics, and goals. Values provide direction that underlie our actions and behaviors, whereas goals are specific things we want to have or achieve. Harris (2009) makes five key points about values: they are in the here and now; they never need to be justified; they often need to be prioritized; they are best held lightly; and they are freely chosen. The first point is that we live according to our values in the present moment; it is never too late to begin living in accordance with our values. Secondly, values are unique and individual to each person and reflect what is meaningful to that person. We don't need to justify our values. The third point is that certain values may take priority over others, depending on the situation or phase of life. Values are best held lightly because when fusion occurs with values, they may begin to feel oppressive and restrictive, like commandments or rules that must be obeyed. Finally, values are freely chosen; we choose to act according to our values because they matter to us.

Committed Action

Committed action means turning values into sustained behaviors toward short-term and long-term goals. Specific action steps build a road toward goals and create a vital, values-based life (Hayes, 2005). Important elements of committed action are the ability to identify barriers and use cognitive defusion, acceptance, and mindfulness to overcome those barriers (Harris, 2009).

These areas of ACT will be discussed in further detail later as they relate to working with youth in the schools. Mindfulness was covered in Chapter 3; here the areas of cognitive defusion, acceptance, self as context, and examining values and related goals will be explored.

Choosing ACT Techniques for Each Youth

Just as most presenting problems have many variations and combinations of symptoms, the ACT techniques selected will vary dependent upon multiple factors, such as the youth's age, developmental level, specific needs and concerns, and background experiences. To move the youth toward psychological flexibility, it is likely you will use multiple metaphors, techniques, and activities. To become overly formulaic in which techniques to use with various presenting concerns could mislead the practitioner. Instead, we recommend that the practitioner try a variety of metaphors and activities with each youth.

Cognitive Defusion

As mentioned in Chapter 1, ACT integrates CBT and mindfulness. In traditional CBT, the process of disrupting attachment to thought is called "distancing" (Beck et al., 1979). Youth are taught to identify, examine, and replace unhelpful thoughts with more helpful, rational thoughts (Merrell, 2008). One key way that ACT differs from traditional CBT is that instead of replacing distorted thoughts, the focus is on altering a person's relationship with their thoughts.

Hayes (2005) writes that it is impossible to stop thinking; there is no pause button on thoughts. This is, in part, adaptive; our mind works to avoid danger and promote survival. It is a process created by evolution to keep us safe. However, this process over time has become a run-away train, absorbing most, if not all of our waking hours, taking us out of the only thing that is real: the present moment. A common metaphor for our thinking minds in Buddhist culture is the "monkey mind," outlined in the following script. The monkey mind begins at a young age. Children may become so engrossed in their thoughts that they lose sight of what is actually happening around them, which can be detrimental to their learning and their social-emotional development. The goal is to reduce children's attachment to their thought processes. This is done through cognitive defusion.

We often become "fused" with our thinking minds, mistaking our thoughts for facts: "If I think it, it must be so." Cognitive defusion is the process of separating ourselves from our thoughts. It involves increasing awareness of thoughts as simply mental events that may or may not represent reality. This reduces attachment to the content of thoughts, thereby creating more acceptance, which introduces more flexibility into the thinking process. The more we are aware of thoughts that arise in our minds, the more openness we can create around our response. This is opposed to trying to eliminate the thought or being flooded by and being reactive to it (Hayes, 2004). In these cases, we don't further evaluate the thought for its utility. Therefore, a goal of ACT is to become more aware of our thoughts in order to disrupt the attachment to them (Hayes, 2005; Tolle, 1999).

As in mindfulness, it can be helpful to first introduce the youth to the concept of cognitive defusion. Following is a sample script that can be used to assist in this.

PRACTITIONER: *Like the hum of an air conditioner in the background, our thoughts often circulate through our minds, doing things like explaining, comparing, predicting, judging, and worrying. Our thinking happens so much that we may not be aware that we are even having thoughts!*

One way of thinking about how our minds work is using the example of a "monkey mind." Our minds swing from thought to thought quickly, without us even being aware of this happening, just like a monkey swings from vine to vine in the jungle. Often, we end up deep in the jungle of our minds, stuck in the story our minds are telling us. When we are so stuck in our thoughts, we do not see what is around us. This is often a reason why we forget if we did things, such as where we parked our bikes at school or if we turned in a paper or not. We are going to talk about and do some things that can help us to let go of the vines and pay more attention to what is around us.

The next section describes a variety of cognitive defusion strategies. A summary of the defusion strategies covered is offered in Table 4.1. Note that imagery may not be as effective with children under the age of 8 or those with cognitive delays; abstract thinking will be more challenging for them. In this case, try the mindfulness and body scan techniques explored in Chapter 3. Because children tend to experience various physical complaints when upset, body scanning can be an appropriate intervention in lieu of the Thought Bubble Meditation or Leaves on the Stream technique. Modifications for younger children are noted in the following exercises, as appropriate. The use of mantras, as described later in this chapter, can also be used with younger children (preschool and older) to assist with loosening negative repetitive thoughts.

Leaves on a Stream Meditation
Ages: 8 years and older
Time: 5+ minutes

A common mindfulness meditation used in ACT to assist with cognitive defusion is the "Leaves on the Stream" (Harris, 2009). When you have a thought during this meditation, you are guided to notice the thought. Then instead of trying to control or change that thought, you imagine putting the thought on a leaf flowing down a stream. A script for this meditation is offered next. A full description of how a practitioner can conduct this meditation with a student is included in Form 4.1. Below is an excerpt of this script.

PRACTITIONER: *We are going to start by taking in some deep, 4x8 breaths. Now, imagine you are sitting by a beautiful, slow-moving stream. Leaves drop down into the stream and float by. Each time a thought pops into your mind, imagine it is on one of the leaves. This can be an image or as written words. Stay beside the stream and allow the leaves to keep flowing by and*

Table 4.1 Summary of cognitive defusion strategies in this chapter.

Strategies	Definitions	Expected Time	Age Range/ Adaptations	Target Process/Outcome
Leaves on a Stream	A meditation using the imagery of placing a thought on a floating leaf on a stream, noticing the thought without further entertaining it, and bringing your attention back to the present moment.	5+ minutes	8 years and older	To notice thoughts without attachment to the thought, thereby bringing the youth back to the present moment. Good for addressing ruminative thoughts.
Thought Bubble Meditation	A meditation that can assist youth in noticing thought without attachment to the thought.	5+ minutes	8 years and older	To notice thoughts without attachment to the thought, thereby bringing the youth back to the present moment. Good for addressing ruminative thoughts.
Sunglasses Metaphor	A metaphor noting that thinking minds are like the lenses of sunglasses: they can change the perspective of how things are seen around us.	5+ minutes	5 years and older	Recognizing how thoughts "color" our experience. Useful when targeting cognitive biases.
Numbers Game	A technique that demonstrates that there is no delete button to use for thoughts.	2+ minutes	8 years and older	Recognizing how we can't make our thoughts disappear. Helpful in addressing ruminative or fused thinking.
"I Am" Labels	A technique to help the youth recognize the power of words.	2+ minutes	8 years and older	To help shift thoughts to allow for more flexibility.
Silly, Sing-Songy Voice	A technique involving changing the tone of the internal message to help create more flexibility in thinking.	3+ minutes	8 years and older	To assist the youth in further defusion of thought. Useful for addressing cognitive fusion.
Milk Technique	An activity involving the repetition of a word, which over time weakens the attachment between the word and its meaning.	3+ minutes	8 years and older	To assist the youth in further defusion of thought. Useful for addressing cognitive fusion.
Physicalizing the Thought/ Emotion	A technique wherein imagery is used to physicalize the thought or feeling, such as giving it color, form, speed, etc.	5+ minutes	5 years and older	To imagine the thought as an external entity. Helpful in supporting students in separating from their thoughts/feelings.
Thought Jar	This activity involves making a "snow globe" that becomes a metaphor for our thinking mind, using a jar, water, and glitter.	10 minutes	5 years and older	To provide a tangible visual representation of our thinking minds.
Tug-of-War	A metaphor depicting the struggle we have with our thoughts, assisting in the idea of "dropping the rope" in the struggle.	2+ minutes	8 years and older	To assist the youth in further defusion of thought.

disappearing. If you notice that you are suddenly somewhere else in your mind, simply notice this has happened and gently bring yourself back to the stream. Stay beside the stream and allow the leaves to keep flowing by, to notice your thoughts without getting caught up in them.

Age Adaptation: This exercise can be adapted into an art activity for younger children. The child writes a word that is troubling to them on a slip of paper and then cuts the paper up into different shapes. The pieces are then pasted onto a pre-cut leaf. This helps decrease the power of the troubling word by making the word meaningless. Then, children can be supported in "letting go" of the thought through activities such as throwing the leaf in the garbage, putting it through the shredder, or flushing it down the toilet.

Thought Bubble Meditation
Ages: 8 years and older
Time: 5+ minutes

The Thought Bubble Meditation can assist youth in noticing a thought without becoming attached to the thought. The following script illustrates the use of this technique.

PRACTITIONER: *We are going to continue our 4x8 breaths today and notice what thoughts come up as we breathe. Ready? Let's take in a deep breath to the count of four, briefly hold it, then let it out to the count of eight.*
YOUTH: (breathing deeply).
PRACTITIONER: *Good. Let's do a few more* (continue to take in 4x8 breaths with the youth). *Now, close your eyes, if you feel comfortable, or lower your gaze. We are going to continue to put our attention on our deep 4x8 breaths and just be right here in the room together. Thoughts may come into our minds as we are breathing. When a thought comes into our minds, we are going to imagine that we put that thought in a bubble, kind of like in a cartoon strip when the characters have thoughts in bubbles above their heads. We are not going to think about the thought more. Instead, we are just going to be aware of the thought and as easily as that thought came into our minds, we will watch that thought float away in the bubble. Let's try that. Notice the thought you are having, place it in a bubble, and then watch that thought float away.*
YOUTH: (continuing to breath and nodding).
PRACTITIONER: *Continue to take in deep breaths to the count of four and let them out to the count of eight. When you notice the next thought come into your mind, place that thought in another bubble, and watch it float away, bringing your awareness back to your deep breathing.*

Age Adaptation: This meditation can be adapted for younger children by making the exercise more concrete. For example, you can have the child draw a comic strip and support them in filling in the "thought bubbles" for the characters. Once the comic strip has been completed, you can prompt the child to "let go" of the thought by discarding it in some fashion. Or you can blow actual bubbles and prompt the child to imagine their thoughts are inside the bubble. Then when the bubble pops, you can coach the youth to bring their attention back to their breath.

Mental Hands
Ages: 8 years and older
Time: 5+ minutes

A second form of imagery to explore attachment to thoughts involves the mind having "mental hands." When thoughts arise in the mind, we have a choice. We can grab onto the thought and create a story for ourselves around it, or we can open our mental hands to the thought and release it into the atmosphere. The following script illustrates this imagery exercise.

PRACTITIONER: *We are going to pretend in our minds we have little hands that hold onto our thoughts. Usually when we have a thought our "mental hands" grab onto the thought, and we pay a lot of attention to the thought. Sometimes our mental hands hold the thought so tightly it's the only thing we focus on, and it makes us not pay attention to the other things around us.*

We are going to practice now as we take in our deep breaths that we are opening our mental hands to these thoughts and letting them float away. Just as easily as thoughts come into our minds, we will open our hands and release them.

Often it works well if the practitioner demonstrates the action of gripping their hands tightly in a fist formation, then opening their hands as they breathe.

Sunglasses
Ages: 5 and older
Time: 5+ minutes

The sunglasses metaphor is intended to help youth understand that their thinking minds are like the lenses of sunglasses: they can change the look of things we see around us. An example of how to introduce this exercise is as follows.

PRACTITIONER: *Today we are going to talk about different shades of sunglasses we might put on, and how they make the world look different. For example, if we put on very dark sunglasses, the world would suddenly appear dark. If we put on red, green, or blue sunglasses, the world around us would have those colors. Our thoughts are like the colors of glasses; they can change or distort how things look which may not be how those things actually are.*

Discuss this with the youth, providing examples of how thoughts can influence how we see things.

Age Adaptation. An adaptation for younger children is to use actual sunglasses with various lens colors, such as yellow, red, and blue. Encourage the child to take them off and on and describe how the world looks different wearing them. Relate this experience to the child's thoughts, and that often what we see is colored by the lens of our thinking minds (e.g., if we had the thought when we wake up, "This is going to be a terrible day." How might this lens taint our experience of the day?).

Numbers Game
Ages: 8 and older
Time: 2+ minutes

This technique introduces youth to the idea that there is no delete button for thoughts (Hayes & Smith, 2005). This becomes important when youth have been actively working on mindfulness and ACT techniques but are bothered because they still have negative thoughts. This technique is more appropriate for older elementary aged students through high school. The script for the numbers game follows.

PRACTITIONER: *It can be hard when we keep remembering thoughts that we are trying to forget. Let's try a quick game, OK?*

YOUTH: *OK.*

PRACTITIONER: *If I were to ask you to say back the following numbers, 1, 2, 3, you would say . . .*

YOUTH: *Um, 1, 2, 3?*

PRACTITIONER: *Right, good. Now, if I were to ask you at the end of our time here together today, 'Hey, what were those 3 numbers I asked you to repeat back to me, what do you think you may remember and say?"*

YOUTH: *1, 2, 3.*

PRACTITIONER: *Good, of course! And tell me this, if in a week I called you up and told you, 'Hey, I have an extra 10,000 dollars in my bank account, and I would love to give it to you if you could try and remember those numbers you repeated during our time together, do you think it is possible you might remember them?"*

YOUTH: *Yes, for sure!!*

PRACTITIONER: *Yes, you probably could. So, do those numbers really mean anything to you besides just being numbers in a row?*

YOUTH: *No, not really.*

PRACTITIONER: *So, if you can remember something that isn't all that meaningful, for a pretty long time, how is it that you think you could forget some of the hurtful things your dad said to you a few years ago?*

YOUTH: (quietly contemplating what the practitioner said).

PRACTITIONER: *So, it isn't the forgetting of the memory or thought that is going to be your key to feeling healthier, it is going to be how much attention and weight you give it; how 'sticky' the thought is and how fused it is in your mind.*

YOUTH: *That makes a lot of sense.*

After playing the numbers game, it is best to move into other defusion techniques, such as Silly, Sing-Songy Voice or Physicalizing the Thought (both introduced next), to assist with creating flexibility in the thinking pattern.

Silly, Sing-Songy Voice:
Ages: 2nd grade and older
Time estimate: 5 minutes

Often, we use an authoritative tone when we repeat painful thoughts to ourselves. Similar to "I am" statements, these negative thoughts can significantly influence how we experience the present moment. It can lead to emotional reactions and behaviors that are unhealthy or inconsistent with what is actually happening. Changing the tone of thoughts can create more flexibility in thinking (Harris, 2009). Before using this technique, develop a good rapport with the youth, so that the silly voice is received in the way it is intended and not as mocking or poking fun. Also, be certain you and the youth have done enough work first on mindfulness and examination of thoughts so that the youth can understand the usefulness of the technique in creating cognitive defusion. The following script illustrates this technique.

PRACTITIONER: *Today we are going to take that thought you have been having, 'No one likes me,' and play with it a little bit. Tell me this, when you have this thought, is it said in a very important voice, like this, (practitioner says this in a deep, authoritative tone) so you really listen to it?*

YOUTH: *Yes, I guess so.*

PRACTITIONER: *Often when we say negative things to ourselves, it is said in an important voice tone that makes us really pay attention to it and believe it. Now tell me this, what would happen if we changed the tone of the voice for this thought?*

YOUTH: *What do you mean?*

PRACTITIONER: *What if, instead of the very important voice tone (practitioner uses deep voice again here), the tone of voice was silly, say, that of Mickey Mouse's voice?*

YOUTH: (Laughs). *Like what?*

PRACTITIONER: *Well, like, instead of 'No one likes me' (practitioner uses deep voice here), we use a Mickey Mouse voice to say, 'No one likes me' (practitioner uses exaggerated, high pitched silly voice).*

YOUTH: (laughs)

PRACTITIONER: *Yes, that's right. It is really hard to pay serious attention to that Mickey Mouse voice. That voice makes it easier to see that it is just a thought we are having, not a real narrative of how things actually are. I would like for you to try this over the next week. When you catch yourself having this thought at school, I want you to change it – repeat it in Mickey Mouse's voice in your head. Reminding yourself it is just a thought you are having, then let yourself come back to the present moment.*

YOUTH: *OK! I am going to do it!*

Milk Technique
Ages: 8 years and older
Time: 3+ minutes

Another defusion technique that is popular with youth is the milk exercise. It was first used in the early 1900s (Tichener, 1916) to decrease the power that certain words hold. It involves saying a word, "milk," repeatedly until the word becomes nonsensical. The repetition over time weakens the attachment between the word and its meaning. In doing this, the literal meaning of the word dissipates; all that is left is a series of sounds that become simply noise. These words then begin to be experienced in a less literal, more flexible way (Greco et al., 2008). An example script of using this technique is below.

PRACTITIONER: *We've been talking a lot about how sad you feel when certain negative thoughts come into your head, like "I'm stupid," right?*

YOUTH: *Yeah.*

PRACTITIONER: *I want to do an exercise with you today that can help you in moments when you're having mean thoughts like that about yourself. First, I want you to think of the word "milk." When you hear that word, what comes to mind? I want you to list out anything that you can think of – other words, images, memories, etc.*

YOUTH: *Well, the first thing I thought of was cows on a dairy farm.*

PRACTITIONER: *Great, what else?*

YOUTH: *I thought of ice cream, pouring milk on my cereal, a milk moustache, and how my little brother gets so mad when my mom makes him drink all of his milk at dinner!*

PRACTITIONER: *Great! Really nice job! Okay, now I want you to do something else. It may seem kind of goofy. I want you to repeat the word "milk" out loud over and over again until I tell you to stop.*

YOUTH: *Milk . . . Milk . . . Milk . . . (continues for 60 seconds)*

PRACTITIONER: *Nice work! What did you notice about the word "milk" as you kept saying it over and over again?*

YOUTH: *Well, at first, it just felt like I was saying the word "milk" but then after I kept saying it, the sounds all started to run together, and it didn't even feel like I was saying a real word anymore!*

PRACTITIONER: *Exactly! Okay, now I want to try it with another word that might have more difficult emotions and memories attached to it. Let's try saying the word "stupid" over and over again.*

Once the youth has gone through this exercise using an emotionally triggering word, the practitioner can highlight how even these types of words become nonsensical over time. You can then encourage the student to use this technique when they notice they are engaging in labeling behaviors, such as calling themselves or others unhelpful or unhealthy names.

Physicalizing the Thought
Ages: 5 years and older
Time: 5+ minutes

A common technique in narrative therapy (Winslade & Monk, 2007) is to "externalize" the problem. This entails taking the thought or feeling and using imagery to physicalize it, such as giving it color, form, and so on. ACT also uses this technique as an aid to create defusion in thinking. Hayes (2005) notes that "when we look at objects external to ourselves, we do not take them to be self-referential" (pg. 137). For example, if we see an object, such as a donut, we do not "become the donut." If, therefore, we are able to externalize a feeling we are having (such as anger), instead of "being angry" we can notice the anger and begin to find ways to distance ourselves from the feeling so that we can better cope with it. The below script illustrates this technique.

PRACTITIONER: *So, you have been talking about how you are anxious this session. Let's play with that thought a little bit. If we were to pull "anxious" out into the room and set it in the empty chair over here, what do you imagine it might look like?*

YOUTH: *Hmmm, look like?*

PRACTITIONER: *Yeah, do you think it may have some shape, or be more of a blob?*

YOUTH: *Oh.* (youth thinks for a bit). *I think it would kind of be like a ball of electricity.*

PRACTITIONER: *Ok, good. What color would it be?*

YOUTH: *Maybe a white color. With orange sparks.*

PRACTITIONER: *OK, and how big would it be?*

YOUTH: *It would take up the whole chair. And maybe as it spins it would grow bigger.*

PRACTITIONER: *Ah, so it would have movement?*

YOUTH: *Yes, for sure. And heat.*

PRACTITIONER: *OK, excellent description. So, it would be a hot ball of white and orange spinning energy that, at times, expands.*

YOUTH: (laughs). *Yeah. That's exactly it!*

Once the youth has externalized the anxiety in this way, the practitioner can now work with the youth on getting some flexibility in their thinking process. The youth no longer "is anxious," but instead can use the language of "when anxiety is in the room," thereby allowing the youth to use breathing and mindfulness techniques to reduce their anxious symptoms as opposed to "being them." This technique of externalization can be used whenever the practitioner notes that youth are using "I am" labels or are particularly flooded by any strong emotion. Because of their abilities to create fantasy characters and stories about life in general, children as young as kindergarten or early elementary, as well as older youth (and even adults) can benefit from this approach. With younger children, it can be helpful to have them draw the externalized feeling with pens or crayons.

Thought Jar
Ages: 5 and older
Time: 10 minutes

This activity involves making a "snow globe" that becomes a metaphor for our thinking mind, using a jar, water, and glitter. The jar and water represent the mind, and the glitter represents the thoughts that we have. The more stirred up our thoughts are in our minds, the more distracted and kinetic the mind is. However, by taking a moment to hold the jar still through mindful awareness, and letting the thoughts settle to the bottom, we can experience more clarity in our minds. The key here is to discuss with the child that we have not gotten rid of the thoughts or altered the thoughts in any way. But we have changed our action around the thoughts, by being still in the present moment, as opposed to continuing to shake up the thoughts in our mind. Form 4.2 contains directions for creating the thought jar. An example script is as follows.

PRACTITIONER: *Today we are going to be making a "Thought Jar." First, we will put glitter of your choice in this clear plastic jar. (Give youth time to add glitter.) Great! I like how many colors you have chosen. Now, we are going to fill the jar with water, leaving a little air at the top. Next, we put a few drops of glycerin in the jar. Now give the jar a few good shakes. As you see, the glitter swirls around. This is like our minds when we are absorbed in thinking. The glitter is like our thoughts, all jumbled and scattered. If we stop, and focus on the present moment, we can settle our minds. Notice that the glitter settles to the bottom when we stop shaking the jar. We haven't gotten rid of our thoughts; like the glitter, they are still there but the water is clearer. When we are quiet and mindful, our thoughts are not stirred up and our mind becomes clear.*

Tug of War
Ages: 8 years and older
Time: 2+ minutes

The struggle we have with our thoughts often carries with it the feeling of having a tug-of-war within our minds. The idea behind this technique is to simply instruct the youth to open their "mental hands" and drop the rope (Hayes, 2004), thereby releasing the power the thought holds on their attention. The below script is an example of how a practitioner could engage a youth in this exercise.

PRACTITIONER: *So, let's think about that thought you are having. It seems to be taking up a lot of your energy during the day, is that right?*
YOUTH: *Yeah.*
PRACTITIONER: *Have you ever played the game "tug-of-war?"*
YOUTH: *Sure!*
PRACTITIONER: *OK, I am guessing that takes a lot of energy too, right? Pulling back and forth and putting a lot of your attention on the task?*
YOUTH: *Oh, for sure! I got sore last time we played that in P.E.*
PRACTITIONER: *Let's imagine now that you are playing tug-of-war in your mind with the thought you keep having of, "No one likes me." You seem to be playing that thought out in your mind a lot, struggling with it, just like you would in a tug-of-war game. You have told me that you feel pretty tired and worn out after having these kinds of thoughts.*
YOUTH: *Yeah, I really do.*
PRACTITIONER: *Ok, now imagine you are playing tug-of-war with someone, and you drop the rope. What would happen?*
YOUTH: *(laughs) The other person pulling on it would fall over!*
PRACTITIONER: *True. How much energy would you put into the game then?*
YOUTH: *None. I would be done.*
PRACTITIONER: *Good, now let's imagine, with that thought you are having of "No one likes me" that you just drop the rope in your mind. No more struggle with the thought. When you notice it, you open your mental hands and tell yourself, "I am dropping the rope and I don't want to play with this thought anymore." Even imagine the scene of how that would look and feel of just dropping the thought.*
YOUTH: *Yeah, then it wouldn't take up so much of my attention. I like that!*

Acceptance and Its Benefits for Youth

Acceptance approaches can be added to mindfulness practices (see Chapter 3) for those youth who are struggling with emotional or behavioral difficulties. As previously mentioned, having thoughts is not the issue; it is the attachment to thoughts that often causes distress. Attachment means wanting reality to be other than what it actually is. Germer (2009) notes that "Pain x Resistance = Suffering" (pg. 15). The pain is the unavoidable discomfort that life brings, such as a loss or change, whereas the resistance is the action we take to eliminate or avoid the pain, such as ruminating on how to make the pain go away, which causes suffering. The opposite of this resistance is acceptance. In ACT, acceptance is moving to reduce attachment to thoughts, feelings, and outcomes. Moving youth toward mindfulness and acceptance can help alleviate their suffering.

Acceptance of thought and situation, as described earlier, is not a giving up or a submission to circumstances. Instead, it is the opposite of experiential avoidance. It brings the individual an active, nonjudgmental awareness and acceptance of the here and now (Hayes, 2004). This awareness gives the individual a clearer picture of what is, as opposed to what is being created in the thinking mind, resulting in an alleviation of suffering.

Techniques for Acceptance

As in most areas of ACT, the use of metaphors and activities can assist the youth in understanding the ideas and the work of acceptance. Acceptance techniques described next are summarized in Table 4.2.

Clipboard Technique:
Ages: 10 years or older
Time: 10+ minutes

There are many variations on this technique; typically, it involves the practitioner using a solid object, such as a clipboard, as a metaphor for the thoughts, feelings, behaviors, or situations with which the youth is struggling (Harris, 2009). The practitioner instructs the youth to do various things with the object to illustrate how they struggle with their current challenges. The youth being "flooded" by the challenge and trying to push away or distract themselves from the challenge are acted out, as is acceptance of the challenge. Following is a script for this technique.

PRACTITIONER: *Today, we are going to do something a little different with the negative thoughts that you have been having. I want you to imagine that this clipboard I am holding represents all of the difficult thoughts, feelings, and memories you have been struggling with. I would like you to take it in your hands and grip it as tightly as you can so that I would not be able to pull it away from you.*

(Practitioner hands clipboard to youth, modeling the gripping action if the youth is unclear as to what to do.)

Good, now I would like you to hold the clipboard up in front of your face so you can't see me anymore. Bring it up close to your face, almost touching

Table 4.2 Summary of acceptance strategies in this chapter.

Strategies	Definitions	Expected Time	Age Range/ Adaptations	Target Process/ Outcome
Clipboard Technique	Using a solid object, such as a clipboard, as a metaphor for the thoughts, feelings, behaviors, or situations with which the youth is struggling.	10 + minutes	10 years and older	Helps youth physicalize their challenge or struggle and allows for a tangible depiction of how to create acceptance around their challenge.
Chinese Finger Trap	Using the toy (either imaginary or an actual finger trap) to help the youth in recognizing the "grip" of the thought and how to have greater awareness of it in order to help "release" the thought from the mind.	3 + minutes	8 years and older	Helps youth physicalize their challenge and allows for a tangible depiction of how to foster acceptance and acknowledgment of the issue instead of struggling with it.
Mantras	Mantras are sayings that can be repeated internally to ourselves as both a form of focused meditation or acceptance.	2+ minutes	5 years and older	To bolster mindfulness and acceptance practices.

your nose. Good. Now, how easy do you think it would be to continue to have a conversation with me while you are holding your thoughts, feelings, and memories so tightly?

YOUTH: *Not easy at all, I can't see you.*

PRACTITIONER: *Yeah. Do you imagine over time you might start to feel distracted or tired gripping that so tightly?*

YOUTH: (laughs) *Yep.*

PRACTITIONER: *And what is your view of the room like holding onto this so tight?*

YOUTH: *I can't see anything but the clipboard.*

PRACTITIONER: *Yes, it is hard to be so absorbed in this stuff and still be able to see clearly what is going on around you. How easy right now would it be to do the things that you have told me that you love to do, like draw, pet your dog, or watch TV? (Fill in activities that are pleasurable for the youth here.)*

YOUTH: *Impossible!*

PRACTITIONER: *Yeah, when we are caught up in difficult thoughts, feelings, and memories, it can be pretty impossible to see or do anything else. OK, you can release the clipboard now.*

YOUTH: (hands clipboard back to practitioner)

PRACTITIONER: *Would it be OK if we tried something else with the clipboard? (Youth nods.) Would it be OK if I came and sat beside you for a moment?*

YOUTH: *Sure.*

PRACTITIONER: *OK, the clipboard still represents the thoughts, feelings, and memories you have been struggling with. What I would like for you to do now is to place both of your hands flat on the clipboard here, and I am going to place my hands on the other side. Now push the clipboard away from you. Push it firmly, but not so hard as to knock me over!*

YOUTH: (Laughs and begins to push on the clipboard. As the youth pushes, the practitioner pushes back to match the intensity.)

PRACTITIONER: *Good, keep pushing. You hate these thoughts, feelings, and memories. You want to get rid of them, to make them go away. So, here you are, trying hard to push this stuff away, but do you notice they are not going anywhere? How easy would it be to continue to have a conversation with me for the rest of our time together while you are pushing like this?*

YOUTH: *Pretty hard! I would get tired, and I don't think I could follow what we are talking about.*

PRACTITIONER: *How easy would it be for you to do the things you enjoy doing, such as draw, pet your dog, or watch TV?* (Fill in activities that are pleasurable for the youth here.)

YOUTH: *Not possible.*

PRACTITIONER: *OK, good. Now go ahead and set the clipboard in your lap. The clipboard still represents the thoughts, feelings, and memories that are hard for you. Do you notice that it is still there?*

YOUTH: *Yeah, I feel it in my lap.*

PRACTITIONER: *Sure, you notice it is still there, but I am guessing there is a lot less effort devoted to it.*

YOUTH: *For sure!*

PRACTITIONER: *How easy would it be now for us to continue to have our conversation?*

YOUTH: *Very easy.*

PRACTITIONER: *And how easy would it be for you to do the things you enjoy doing, such as draw, pet your dog, or watch TV?* (Fill in activities that are pleasurable for the youth here.)

YOUTH: (pretends to pet a dog). *Much easier.*

PRACTITIONER: *So, no longer is it the only thing you can see* (practitioner holds an imaginary clipboard up in front of their face), *and no longer are you trying to get rid of these thoughts, feelings, and memories* (practitioner demonstrates the pushing motion). *Instead, you notice that they are still there, but you are devoting less energy toward them, just noticing them without attaching to them. This helps you see things around you more clearly and gives you more energy to do the things you love to do.*

YOUTH: *Yeah, I see what you are saying.*

In later sessions, the clipboard metaphor can be referred to when the practitioner notices that the youth is either feeling flooded by their thoughts, feelings, or memories, trying to distract themselves, or push these experiences away. Children in later elementary school through young adulthood can benefit from this activity, though the concept may be too abstract for younger children.

Chinese Finger Trap
Ages: 8 years or older
Time: 3+ minutes

Another common metaphor for acceptance used in ACT is the Chinese finger trap (Hayes & Smith, 2005). If the practitioner notes that the youth is struggling with a repetitive thought, this strategy can help the youth recognize the grip of the thought and how to release the thought from the mind. The below script illustrates this technique.

PRACTITIONER: (holding an actual finger trap, which can be given to the youth at the end of the session as a reminder in between sessions of the grasp that thoughts have on us) *Place your fingers in the toy finger trap. Good. Now, try to remove your fingers. Do you notice the more you struggle to get your fingers out of the trap, the greater it holds on? Now, relax your fingers, perhaps even easing them together a bit. Notice how the trap releases and your fingers are free! The mind is also like this: the more we struggle with our thoughts, the greater their hold. However, once we use mindfulness and breathwork to stop struggling and just allow our thoughts to come and go, we can be released from them.*

Mantras
Ages: 3 years and older
Time: 2+ minutes

Mantras are sayings that can be repeated internally as a form of focused meditation. For example, a child with separation anxiety can repeat the following saying throughout the day, "I am safe here." or "I am brave." or "My mom will pick me up soon." These mantras would allow thoughts to shift away from negative rumination to the present moment (Holland et al., 2017). Acceptance can also be fostered through mantras, such as by repeating, "This situation is hard, but I am strong and calm in the face of it." or "I see the struggle I have, and I can remain calm and healthy in this moment." Mantras can also be coupled with 4x8 breathing. Following are some examples of this pairing of techniques.

> *Breathing in I am calm, breathing out I am relaxed.*
> *Breathing in I am safe, breathing out my needs are met.*
> *Breathing in I am loved, breathing out I am cared for.*

The above mantras would be internally practiced (repeating the thought again and again) as the youth is slowly breathing in and out. What mantra is used will be dependent on the youth and the presenting concern. Sometimes it can be helpful to write down the mantra for the youth so that they can remember it and carry it with them or post it somewhere noticeable (e.g., on the back of their bedroom door, taped inside their school binder, etc.). Mantras can be helpful for youth throughout their development; even preschool children are able to internalize healthy self-talk and use breathing techniques.

Self-as-Context

As discussed previously, self-as-context is essentially "awareness of our own awareness" (Harris, 2009). It is the "I" of our observing self. We may say, "I am depressed." or "I am anxious." These "I Am" labels can be very powerful, saying simply we ARE these conditions. Now consider how we refer to our physical health. We would not say, "I am the flu," or "I am cancer" when discussing our medical condition. Instead, we would say something along the lines of, "I have symptoms of the flu." The idea of *having symptoms of*, as opposed to *being the condition*, allows for some flexibility in the ability to change, alter, or treat the condition. Self-as-context is the part of the self "doing the noticing" and can, therefore, facilitate cognitive defusion and acceptance. Once we understand the concept of the observing self, we can better understand how to simply observe and accept thoughts and feelings (Harris, 2009; Hayes et al., 2012). Techniques for increasing this noticing of self are offered next.

"I Am" Labels
Ages: 8 years and older
Time: 2+ Minutes

Discuss with the child the idea of "I Am" labels, as discussed in the previous section, and how powerful these can be. The only thing that we definitively know is that we are human. Almost everything else is alterable. This shift in thinking puts emotional distance between the label and the experience of it in the moment, thereby helping our awareness of ourselves (Hayes, 2004). An example of how to describe this concept to a youth is below.

PRACTITIONER: *We are going to talk about "I am" statements today. These are thoughts we have that start with the words, "I am." For example, if we have blonde hair, we may say "I am blonde." However, if we are blonde and we want to change our hair color to brown, we can change our hair color; if we have a headache, we can take some medicine to make it better. One of the only things we really are is human!*

When we have the thought, "I am anxious." we can make changes with that too! We can change our thinking around it. Instead of "I AM anxious." we can tell ourselves, "I am having the thought that I am anxious. It is just a thought, like any other thought. Now I will focus on what can help me to feel calm." In this way the thought becomes less defining and opens up other possibilities for how to make changes or feel better.

The "Noticing Part" of Ourselves
Ages: 8 years and older
Time: 2+ Minutes

One way of helping youth to understand the part of ourselves that is "doing the observing" is to name the noticing part of ourselves (Harris, 2009). For example, as we notice things going on around us, it's the observer part of ourselves that is doing this action. Following is a script to help the youth understand this "noticing part" of ourselves.

PRACTITIONER: *The "noticing part" of ourselves is the part that does the observing. For example, if you're eating peppermints, you are using a part of you that we call the mouth; and if you are smelling flowers, you are using a part of you that we call the nose. And when you are doing all this noticing, that's a part of ourselves for which we don't have a word in everyday language. For our work, we will call this the "noticing part" of you.*

Letter to Older, Wiser Self
Ages: 8 years and older
Time: 10+ Minutes

Another exercise that can help to increase self-awareness as related to self-as-context is to have the youth write a letter to themselves from the perspective of their older, wiser self. This is a twist on compassionate letter writing, wherein you imagine writing a letter from the perspective of a caring friend toward yourself (Ackerman, 2017). In the Letter to Older, Wiser Self, the youth is forced into the observer-self role as they are reflecting back on their life, giving words of wisdom and encouragement, from a future-self perspective. To introduce this exercise, you can use the following script.

PRACTITIONER: *Today you are going to write a letter from your older, wiser self to yourself right now. Imagine that your 60 or 80-year-old self is writing to you. What do you imagine they would say about you in this moment? What words of encouragement or greater perspective do you think your older, wiser self could offer? If you like, you can tell me the things that you think your older self would say and I can write down what you are saying if that makes it easier.*

Note that this exercise can also be given as something that the youth completes between sessions.

Values

Identifying Values and Values-Based Goals

As described earlier, values are chosen life directions and are a key area in ACT that furthers psychological flexibility. Values are not the same as goals, but ideally, they inform our goals and intentions. People are most motivated to follow through on goals that align with their values. The following section offers strategies for values exploration and mindful goal setting (Table 4.3). To make this process more concrete for younger children, consider using tangible objects, such as cards with pictures that represent different values, from which the youth can select. Once values have been selected, the practitioner should then support the youth in developing simple goals.

Values List
Ages: 8 years and older
Time: 10+ minutes

One way to determine what the youth values is through creation of a values list (Harris, 2009). Some of the most commonly held values for youth fall in the following areas: family relationships; peer friendships; education; hobbies and leisure activities; spirituality; citizenship; and health/physical well-being (Hayes, 2005). Other areas can be added when appropriate (see Form 4.3). The following script illustrates how to describe this exercise.

PRACTITIONER: *Today we are going to talk about the areas of your life that you value. Some areas that clients tell me they value are their family, their friendships, their education, their hobbies and things they do to relax and have*

Table 4.3 Summary of values and goals strategies in this chapter.

Strategies	Definitions	Expected Time	Age Range/ Adaptations	Target Process/ Outcome
Values List	The creation of a values list with the youth.	10 + minutes	8 years and older	Helps youth to identify their core values.
Eightieth Birthday Party	An activity wherein the youth imagines three people who, at the youth's eightieth birthday, will stand up and give a speech about the youth, including what the youth stood for in their life. The descriptors that are included in the "speeches" are often the areas the youth most values.	10 + minutes	10 years and older	Helps youth to identify their core values
Roadmap to Success	This activity aids youth in creating short-term to long- term goal setting, with youth writing next to the "road signs" actions that will help them meet their values-based goals.	15+ minutes	8 years and older	Assists youth in setting short-term to long-term goals.

fun, their spirituality, their community or country, and their health and physical well-being. We are going to talk about some examples and specific circumstances for each of these areas (proceed to do this with the youth).

Now we will rank the seven values by their importance to you, ordering them 1 through 7. This will help us to see what is most important to you at this time so that we can make some short-term to long-term goals based on these areas (see Roadmap to Success activity).

Note that the values can also be written on index cards and manually ordered to create a hierarchy of those that are most important to the youth at that time.

Eightieth Birthday Party
Ages: 10 years and older
Time: 10+ minutes

The eightieth birthday party is a technique that can help the youth further explore what they value (Harris, 2009) via the perspectives of people who knew them throughout their life. The descriptions included in the speeches are often the areas the youth most values. Below is an example of how to facilitate this exercise.

PRACTITIONER: *Today we are going to have you imagine three people who will stand up at your eightieth birthday and give a speech about you, including what you stood for in your life. This is your fantasy, so you can include people who may not still be alive at the time of this party, such as your parents or grandparents, or who may not exist in this moment, such as a future life partner, co-worker, spouse, or child. One by one, these three people will say a few sentences about you* (go through each person and note what they would say about the youth).

    The things you shared with me in these speeches are likely things that you value in your life or things you want to accomplish. Let's talk about that.

Form 4.4 contains more details about this technique. The practitioner can discuss with the youth what specific actions and behaviors can be taken to support these values listed from the "speeches." Together you can formulate goals to support the values identified as most important.

Road Map to Success
Ages: 8 years and older
Time: 15+ minutes

The Road Map to Success can aid youth in setting short-term or long-term goals. On the map, the youth will write next to the "road signs" actions that will help them meet their goals that are aligned with their values, as found through the 80th Birthday Party and/or the Values List activities. An example of how to support youth through this activity is as follows.

PRACTITIONER: (Hand the youth Handout 5.3 from Chapter 5.) *Today we are going to make a roadmap to your goals. First, choose one value that you rated highly on your values list (Form 4.3). Let's write that down here. Now, let's discuss goals that would support that value. (Discuss with youth.) Great, now we are going to think of actions that would move you toward your values-based goals.*

The practitioner can give an example. If the student highly values "academics" then to, "improve as a student" is a likely goal. From this goal, a possible first action step that can move the student toward the goal is, "organize my backpack." A medium-term action might be, "use my planner to check off assignments and remember upcoming tests over the next two weeks." A longer-term action might be, "finish papers before deadlines and study for tests over the weekends." These actions could all be added to Handout 5.3's road signs 1 through 5, respectively.

Setting Values-Based Intentions in Meditation

Setting intentions for meditation is essentially determining what the focus of the meditation practice will be for that day. This can vary from day to day, and even hourly. The following is a brief list of possible intentions that can be discussed with the youth that they may want to focus on:

Health
Calm
Happiness
Peace
Productivity

There are various ways intentions can be set, including using the intention as a focused meditation (see earlier section of this chapter), asking the youth what intention they would like to focus on that day and selecting techniques that can help to support that intention. For example, if their response was "calm," then the work could focus on breath and bodywork, with perhaps some cognitive defusion work for troublesome thoughts. Intentions can also be used as a form of goal setting in therapy.

Relapse Prevention: When Setbacks Happen

In mindfulness and ACT, as in most practices, setbacks are likely to happen. You can work with the youth to prepare them for setbacks, also known as relapse prevention. Perhaps they forget to use their mindfulness skills, or they once again begin to feel overwhelmed by their thoughts or a specific negative experience. Bringing the possibility of setbacks to the youth's attention can be helpful. Make sure they know that they can practice the tools learned in mindfulness and ACT to get back on track. Four metaphors, summarized in Table 4.4, can assist the discussion of setbacks: the swamp metaphor, passengers on the bus, the flip side of the paper, and mountain climbing metaphor.

The Swamp Metaphor
Ages: 8 years and older
Time: 5+ minutes

When using the swamp metaphor (Harris, 2009), the practitioner compares the youth's progress toward their goal to a hike toward the peak of a mountain. Often on hikes, we encounter unexpected circumstances, such as a swamp. We have to decide: turn back and give up, stay

Table 4.4 Summary of ACT relapse prevention strategies in this chapter.

Strategies	Definitions	Expected Time	Age Range/ Adaptations	Target Process/Outcome
The Swamp Metaphor	The practitioner compares the youth's progress toward their goal to a hike toward the peak of a mountain, helping youth make decisions when setbacks happen, such as turning back and giving up, staying stuck in the swamp, or moving through it.	5 + minutes	8 years and older	To provide the youth with a tangible image of grit and resilience toward goals.
Passengers on the Bus	This metaphor involves the imagery of the youth as the bus driver, and the passengers as their thoughts, with the driver continuing to move toward their destination – that is, their goal or value – even when the passengers are unruly or negative.	10 + minutes	10 years and older	Imagining or acting out disruptive thinking and practicing acceptance as the youth moves toward the identified goals.
Flip Side of the Paper	This technique involves the youth using one side of a piece of paper to write about a challenge they are having, and the other side of the paper to write the values area that challenge is related to, thereby determining if the value is important enough to the youth to shift their attachment to the challenge and persevere.	5+ minutes	12 years and older	To help the youth identify if the challenge is over-riding their core value. To help the youth to either make a determined change in their life, or to change their attachment around the challenge.
Mountain Climbing Metaphor	A useful metaphor for setbacks using the simple imagery of climbing a mountain.	5+ minutes	5 years and older	To help the youth more reasonably assess their setback or challenge and see that it does not have to be couched as a failure, but instead as a detour on their path, one that may lead to even more progress in the end.

stuck in the swamp, or move through it. The following script shows how to use this metaphor when supporting a student through challenges on the way to completing a goal.

PRACTITIONER: *We have been talking a lot the last few weeks about the goals that you are working on. Sometimes as we move toward our goals, problems can crop up. We usually don't have control over these problems, but we can control how we react to them. Let's imagine that your goal is to make it to the top of a mountain peak that you have always wanted to climb. Can we take a few moments right now, take a few deep breaths, and imagine this mountain?*

YOUTH: Sure. (Youth closes eyes and takes in some deep breaths.)

PRACTITIONER: *OK, so imagine you are walking along your path toward the mountain, and you are feeling pretty good about your progress. The sun is out, and the air feels good.*

YOUTH: *Yeah, I like hiking.*

PRACTITIONER: *Now imagine right as you get up to the base of the mountain, right before you are going to make that final climb up, you stumble upon a swamp. This swamp encircles the entire mountain, so there is no way to avoid it. It's gooey and green and you hadn't expected it to be there at all. It is a big surprise! So now you have to decide what to do. Do you throw your hands up and give up on your goal?*

YOUTH: *No way!*

PRACTITIONER: *OK, well, would you wade into the swamp and hang out in it. Swim around and decide to stay in it. Perhaps do the backstroke?*

YOUTH: (laughs) *Gross, no!*

PRACTITIONER: *There is one other choice you can make. You can tell yourself, "Well, here is a swamp. This is not going how I thought it would, and I had not expected this swamp. But I will have to accept that it is here, and I will move through it without getting stuck or giving up on my goal."*

YOUTH: *Yeah, OK, I see where you are going with it.*

PRACTITIONER: *Yes, often as we move toward our goals, we encounter swamps. It's not what we expected, nor what we wanted, but we can just accept that they are there and move through them so that we can be on our way.*

This technique can be used with almost all ages. Incorporate visuals or an art project for younger children. For example, use finger paints to create the goal on the hill and the swamp surrounding it.

Passengers on the Bus
Ages: 10 years and older
Time: 10+ minutes

The "passengers on the bus" metaphor involves the imagery of the youth as the bus driver, and the passengers as their thoughts. The idea here is that even though the passengers may be noisily shouting and chattering in the background, the driver can continue to move toward their destination (i.e., their values-based goal; Hayes et al., 2012).

A script for this is included in Chapter 5. Describe the scene to the youth, even role playing the situation with them. The practitioner takes on the role of the driver moving toward the goal and the youth takes on the role of the negative or unhelpful thoughts (e.g., "Discuss how this can be applied to any goal such as studying for a math test. The unruly passengers might be thoughts like, "You are going to fail!," and "Why even bother studying?").

Age Adaptation: For elementary-aged children, have them draw a bus on a piece of paper, including a driver moving toward the goal ahead on a road, and the passengers in the back shouting negative thoughts.

A further description of how this exercise can be used when working with groups is offered in Chapter 5.

Flip Side of the Paper
Ages: 12 years and older
Time: 5+ minutes

The flip side of the paper technique is especially appropriate for older children and adolescents. This exercise helps to clarify if the value-based goal is still important to be working on for the youth, even when a challenge or problem arises. It can help to determine if the youth should continue toward their values-based goal considering the obstacle or if they perhaps need to change direction in what they are working toward (Harris, 2009). The following script illustrates how to engage youth in this exercise.

PRACTITIONER: (Give the youth a piece of paper.) *On one side of the paper, write about a challenge you are having, such as an argument with your friend or a tricky homework assignment. Then, on the other side of the paper, write the values area that challenge is related to. For example, if you wrote about the argument, then the value area would be friendship. If you wrote about your homework, the value area would be education. OK, now if I could grant you the power, would you get rid of the challenge, tearing up the paper and throwing it away? To do so, you would have to give up both sides of the paper: you cannot have one side of the paper, the challenges, without the other, the value.*

Note here, if the youth says the value is important, then focus your discussion on the value and suggest that the youth use various learned techniques to approach the challenge area (such as acceptance, mindfulness, or cognitive defusion practices). If the youth wants to get rid of the paper altogether, you can initiate an exploration of values in order to further understand the youth's inner world.

Mountain Climbing Metaphor
Ages: 5 years and older
Time: 5+ minutes

A useful metaphor for setbacks can be the simple imagery of climbing a mountain. Use the mountain climbing analogy to help youth more reasonably assess a setback or challenge.

PRACTITIONER: *Mountain climbers often experience some setbacks as they are going up the mountain. The adjustments they make, such as taking a step back, taking in a deep breath, and reassessing their footing, can give surer stability and help move them even higher toward their goal. Setbacks do not have to be a failure; they can be seen as detours on the path that may lead to even more progress in the end. Challenges can actually present us with an opportunity to use our new skills.*

For younger children, the use of a visual can be helpful, such as the Mountain Handout in Chapter 5.

Case Examples

Joshua, Age 10
Presenting Concern: Anger Management Problems and Depression

Joshua (he/him/his) is a fifth grader referred by his teacher and grandparent (his legal guardian) for aggressive acting out behaviors, including yelling at and pushing peers and some destruction of property. When he is caught engaging in these acts, Joshua often tells others that he is the "bad kid" and states "no one cares about me." Grandparent and teacher interviews suggest Joshua is suffering from low self-esteem and some depressive symptoms, in addition to his aggressive externalizing behaviors. The practitioner decided to use ACT with Joshua, including the mindfulness practices overviewed in Chapter 3, given his age and presenting concerns.

Joshua presented to the practitioner as bright but somewhat unmotivated to be in counseling. He saw the issues he was having as "everyone else's problem" and that people were "against him." The practitioner decided to begin with psychoeducation about how our bodies and minds work such as: scanning the environment for threat; focusing on the negative; and the fight, flight, freeze response. Joshua immediately could relate to this and gave examples from his own life of these experiences. In the second session, the practitioner used some 4x8 breathing skills (see Chapter 3) to initially assist Joshua in reducing his reactivity and nervous system response, incorporating the thought bubble meditation over the next few sessions.

In the third session, the practitioner worked with Joshua on identifying goals based on what he values, as discovered by completing the Values List (Form 4.3) and the Roadmap to Success (Handout 5.3) handouts. Joshua identified that "happiness" and "relationships" were primary values of importance to him. It was decided that a primary goal would be to learn more effective ways to cope with his anger. In the fourth session, the practitioner used the Sunglasses Metaphor to help Joshua further understand how the way we think taints and changes the way we see things. Joshua noted that he was presuming that others were "out to get him," and this led him to feel angry even when others had done nothing to provoke his anger. In session five, the practitioner worked on physicalizing Joshua's "anger," asking him how he feels internally in his body when anger is in the room. Joshua acknowledged that his muscles grow tight; he notices a quickened heart rate and his face becomes flush. In further physicalizing anger, Joshua drew out what anger looks like in the room – a red, hot spinning ball of fire with jagged teeth. The practitioner then discussed ways of using the 4x8 breathing to reduce this reactivity in his body. Acceptance techniques such as the Chinese Finger Trap were also used to help release the grip of anger.

In the final session, the Passengers on the Bus metaphor was used to assist Joshua in moving toward his goals, while simply acknowledging but not attaching to the voice of anger ("just give up" and "they will never like you"). Finally, setbacks were discussed using the Swamp Metaphor and the Mountain Climbing Metaphor. Joshua was encouraged to move toward his goals, anticipating there may be a few diversions in his path, but he can accept them and continue to make progress.

At follow-up, Joshua's teacher and grandparent both noted a decrease in aggressive acting out behaviors and increased positive mood. Joshua reported that he had strengthened several relationships with his classmates and felt happier at school, with anger having less control over his mood and relationships.

Lucy, Age 17
Presenting Concern: Anxiety

Lucy (she/her/hers) is a junior in high school, self-referred for anxiety and occasional panic attacks. According to both Lucy and her mother, Lucy has been worried about the college admissions process and has become hyper-focused on her school performance and grades, leading to perfectionistic thinking in this area. The practitioner decided to use ACT with Lucy.

In the initial session, the practitioner provided psychoeducation to Lucy about how thoughts are like tigers, with her thoughts leaping at her and activating her nervous system, just like a real threat in the room. In session two, the practitioner led Lucy through some 4x8 breathing and introduced Lucy to the Leaves on the Stream meditation (Form 5.1) in order to support her in defusing from her perfectionistic thoughts.

In session three, the practitioner used the Eightieth Birthday Party (Form 4.4) to help Lucy identify what she values in her life. Lucy noted across all three speakers at her party that she valued family, community, and taking on academic or career-oriented challenges. No one said she had to be "perfect" in order to achieve great things. The practitioner took those values and helped Lucy create some short-term to long-term goals using the Roadmap to Success (Form 4.5). In session four, Lucy discussed with the practitioner her fears of not getting into college, "failing" in life, and her need to be "perfect." The practitioner noted that Lucy used a great deal of "I am" language (e.g., I am anxious; I am a failure). These "I am" labels were discussed and reframed as, "I am having the thought that . . . ." The practitioner then used the Clipboard Technique to help Lucy recognize the struggle she has been in with these anxious thoughts. She was encouraged to acknowledge her thoughts without having them flood her or feeling she needed to push the thoughts away.

In the fifth session, Lucy was frustrated because she was continuing to have anxious thoughts. She was under the impression that through this work, the thoughts would naturally diminish. The practitioner discussed how her fused, perfectionistic thinking had created a situation where she feels stuck. The practitioner played The Numbers Game with Lucy to help her recognize that there is no delete button on thoughts; instead, the goal is to decrease her attachment to her thoughts.

In the sixth and final session, the practitioner used the Passengers on the Bus metaphor to help Lucy steer toward her goals, even when the "passengers" were dissuading her (e.g., "You will never make it! You are not good enough!"). Lucy said she felt empowered thinking of herself as the bus driver and thoughts as just noisy passengers behind her. Finally, the Swamp Metaphor was discussed in the context of her moving toward her goals, while having realistic expectations that setbacks were likely to occur along the way.

At follow-up, Lucy rated her anxiety as significantly lower than when she started the sessions with the practitioner. Her mother agreed; she has noticed Lucy appearing calmer and less reactive toward her schoolwork and college applications.

Conclusion

The incorporation of ACT and mindfulness work can be a powerful addition to your therapeutic toolbox when working with youth. ACT techniques can build awareness of children's thinking minds and help to further ground them in the present moment. Youth are often not aware of the impact their thinking has on their feelings and behavior. Yet this awareness can be especially important in the school setting where it is necessary for youth to perform academically, while also navigating peer and teacher relationships. The latter are critical in the social and emotional development of children. This chapter overviewed acceptance practices that can be used with individual youth in the school setting. The next chapters describe how mindfulness and ACT techniques can be used when working with school-based groups.

Form 4.1

Leaves on a Stream
Materials Needed: See age adaptation below
Age Adaptations: 8 and older, see age adaptation below

It is best when starting this exercise to first engage the youth in some 4x8 breaths, as depicted in Chapter 3.

Script:

As you continue to take in your deep, four by eight breaths, I want you to imagine a beautiful, slow-moving stream. The water is flowing over rocks, around trees, and through a valley. Once in a while, a big leaf drops into the stream and floats away down the river. Imagine you are sitting beside the stream, watching the leaves float by.

Now become conscious of your thoughts. Each time a thought pops into your mind, imagine that it is written on one of those leaves. If it is easier, imagine placing the image or words from your mind on the leaf. The goal in this activity is to stay beside the stream and allow the leaves on the stream to keep flowing by. Don't try to make the stream go faster or slower, and don't try to change what thoughts are placed on the leaves.

If you notice you are all of a sudden mentally somewhere else, and the stream or leaves have disappeared, just notice that this has happened, and gently bring yourself back to the stream and noticing your thoughts on the leaves.

Practitioner note: Allow pauses in the script to allow time for the youth to imagine the stream without interruption. Small prompts, such as "as you take in this next deep breath and let it out, notice the flow of the stream and the leaves holding your thoughts as they make their way along," can be offered to help the youth refocus and continue in the imagery. Allow three to four minutes of practice with this exercise, depending on the youth's ability to participate in this exercise. Debrief with the youth if the exercise was challenging in any way, if they noticed they lost track of the stream and began thinking about other things, and how continuing to practice this will allow the youth to do better over time in allowing the stream to flow.

Age Adaptation: This activity can be adapted to be an art activity, wherein the youth writes a word that is troubling to them on a small slip of paper, then cuts that paper up into different shapes and pastes the shapes onto a pre-cut leaf. This allows the youth to take a word that is powerful to them and to decrease its power via making the word meaningless. Finally, support the youth in "letting go" of the thought by throwing it in the garbage can, putting it through a paper shredder, or flushing it down the toilet.

Adapted from Harris (2009).

Form 4.2

Thought Jar
Materials Needed:

- Clear glass or plastic jars
- Glitter of various colors
- Water
- Glycerin or corn syrup

Age Adaptations: None, can be used with ages 5 and older

Directions:

- Instruct youth to put glitter of their choosing in their jars.
- Fill the youth's jars with water, dropping in a few drops of glycerin/ corn syrup, leaving a little air at the top.

Script:

Now that you have your glitter and water in your jar, go ahead and give it a few good shakes. See how the glitter is swirling around in your jars. This is like how our minds become when we are absorbed in our thinking minds. The glitter is like our thoughts, all jumbled and scattered in our minds. If we stop and become quiet, we settle our minds. Notice that the glitter settles to the bottom of the jar when we stop shaking the jar. We haven't deleted the thoughts, but instead have allowed them to settle. Your thoughts are still there, as the glitter is still there. When we allow the jar to sit without shaking it, the glitter settles to the bottom and the water is clear. When we become quiet and mindful, our thoughts are not stirred up and our minds become clear.

Form 4.3

Values List
Materials Needed:

- Handout
- Pen

Age Adaptations: May need to define or give examples of the following values; 10 years or older

Values List Handout

Rank order the below, 1–7, in order of most importance in your life. Give an example of one way you can support this value through something you can do.

Rank	Value	Example of an Action You Can Take
____	Family relationships	
____	Peer friendships	
____	Academics	
____	Hobbies and leisure activities	
____	Spirituality	
____	Citizenship	
____	Health and physical well-being	

Form 4.4

Eightieth Birthday Party
Materials Needed: None
Age Adaptations: Language used in script may need adjusting to
   youth's developmental level

The Eightieth Birthday Party is a technique to assist in clarifying values. The following script is adapted from Harris (2009).

Script:

Today we are going to have you imagine your eightieth birthday party. Take a moment to imagine the scene, with the decorations, the food, and the music. Now imagine that three different people stand up to make speeches about you. This is your fantasy birthday party, so these people can be anyone you want, including people who have already died, such as a grandparent or parent you don't think will still be alive when you turn eighty, or a future child, boss, or best friend. This is your fantasy, so include anyone whom you truly care about, OK?

Now imagine the first person you have chosen gets up and makes a short speech about you, just a few sentences. The speech will be about what you stand for in life and what you mean to them. Go ahead and take a few moments to think about that and tell me what they will say.

(Practitioner allows some time for the youth to think about this, and share what the first person would say. The practitioner then repeats the instruction for the two other people who will give speeches, allowing time for the youth to reflect and respond).

The things that you shared with me that would be included in these speeches are likely things that you value in your life or things you want to accomplish. Let's talk about that, and how knowing these values and goals can be helpful to you in this moment.

References

Ackerman, C. (2017, December 5). *9 self-compassion exercises & worksheets for increasing compassion.* PositivePsychology.com. https://positivepsychology.com/self-compassion-exercises-worksheets/

Beck, A. T., Rush, A. J., Shaw, B. F., & Emery, G. (1979). *Cognitive therapy of depression.* Guilford Press.

Germer, C. (2009). *The mindful path to self-compassion: Freeing yourself from destructive thoughts and emotions.* Guilford Press.

Greco, L. A., Barnett, E. R., Blomquist, K. K., & Gevers, A. (2008). Acceptance, body image, and health in adolescence. In L. A. Greco & S. C. Hayes (Eds.), *Acceptance & mindfulness treatments for children and adolescents: A practitioner's guide* (pp. 187–214). New Harbinger Publications.

Harris, R. (2009). *ACT made simple: A quick start guide to ACT basics and beyond.* New Harbinger Publication.

Hayes, S. C. (2004). Acceptance and commitment therapy. In S. C. Hayes, V. M. Follette, & M. M. Linehan (Eds.), *Mindfulness and acceptance: Expanding the cognitive-behavioral tradition* (pp. 1–29). Guilford Press.

Hayes, S. C., & Smith, S. (2005). *Get out of your mind and into your life: The new acceptance and commitment therapy.* New Harbinger Publications.

Hayes, S. C., Strosahl, K. D., & Wilson, K. G. (2012). *Acceptance and commitment therapy: An experiential approach to behavior change* (2nd ed.). Guilford Press.

Holland, M. L., Hawks, J., & Gimpel Peacock, G. (2017). *Emotional and behavioral problems of young children: Effective interventions in the preschool and kindergarten year* (2nd ed.). Guilford Press.

Merrell, K. W. (2008). *Helping students overcome depression and anxiety: A practical guide* (2nd ed.). Guilford Press.

Tichener, E. B. (1916). *A text-book of psychology.* Macmillan.

Tolle, E. (1999). *The power of now: A guide to spiritual enlightenment.* New World Library.

Winslade, J. M., & Monk, G. D. (2007). *Narrative counseling in schools: Powerful & brief* (2nd ed.). Corwin Press.

5 Mindfulness and ACT Strategies for Small Group Work

Roadmap to Chapter 5:
   This chapter overviews considerations for running an eight-week small group program using mindfulness and ACT practices. Specifically, it covers:

- ideas for setting up the group
- developmental adaptations
- a comprehensive eight-week group curriculum

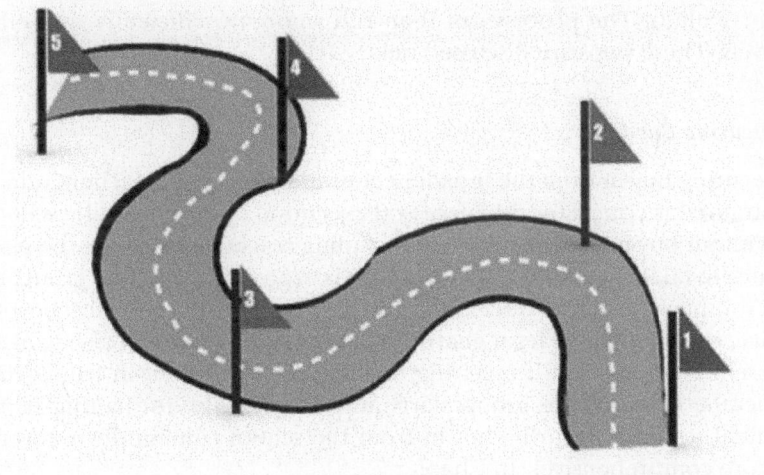

The advantages of running groups in schools is well documented (Cooley, 2009). Early intervention groups have been found to have the most promising results (Gerrity & Delucia-Waack, 2006). A meta-analysis of group treatments with youth aged 4–18 found that group treatments were significantly more effective for children than wait-list and placebo control interventions (Hoag & Burlingame, 2009).

DOI: 10.4324/9781003318101-5

There are many advantages to using a group therapy format in a school setting. From a practical perspective, it maximizes treatment accessibility in terms of time- and cost-effectiveness. Instead of providing individual counseling appointments to six children, all six can be served in the same hour. A group format also provides increased opportunities for social connections, as well as the ability to harness the power of peer influence in a structured group setting. Children are oftentimes more receptive to things their peers say, in comparison to what an adult may suggest. In fact, research has demonstrated that peers offering advice, encouragement, and attention can be powerful contributors to change. Furthermore, many of the concerns that students have are focused on social issues and the group format can be used to address these social problems.

This chapter will first address how to set up a small group in a school setting. It will then detail an eight-session curriculum for a group on mindfulness and ACT practices.

Getting Started

Getting a group started in the schools can initially seem daunting. Key steps are securing proper buy-in from all stakeholders, setting up the parameters of the group to ensure best practices, and using a detailed curriculum. The process can then run smoothly, efficiently, and effectively. These steps are discussed next.

Securing Buy-In

Securing buy-in from the broader community (parents, teachers, administrators) is critical for the successful execution of a group in the schools. Without buy-in from the school, including teachers, there may be resistance to taking students away from the classroom to attend the group; the result may be lack of referrals to the group. As with any counseling service, consent from a legal guardian is essential. You should also gain the assent from the youth receiving the service. Secure buy-in from group members before the group starts and through the formatting of the initial sessions. Securing buy-in from the school community is covered more comprehensively in Chapter 7.

Setting

The physical setting for groups will vary depending on the number of group members and the activities that are to be run in the group. We recommend that the physical space be in a room small enough to facilitate a close and intimate group experience, while large enough to accommodate movement and creative activities. Preferably the group can sit in a circle or semicircle format. It should be as free from distractions as possible (Haen & Aronson, 2016).

Selection of Members

Once consent has been obtained from the legal guardians, it can be helpful to do a short, in-person screening with the youth selected for the group. This is to be certain the selected members' presenting concerns are homogenous enough so that there are no significant outliers (e.g., their needs do not match the rest of the members), to be sure each is a good match socially for the group, and to be certain the student has buy-in and agrees to participate.

During the individual screening, the group facilitator should explain the purpose of the group to the youth, along with group expectations, such as confidentiality and active participation in the sessions. Gather additional information about the challenges the youth is currently experiencing (e.g., difficulties concentrating, depressed mood). Do they often feel stressed? Do they, at times, have challenges in their relationships with peers, teachers, or parents? These questions can help the facilitator better understand the referral. Be sure to also inquire about the youth's strengths, talents, interests, and hobbies. These questions can help to further rapport and create buy-in.

Screening also allows the practitioner to determine if the youth would benefit from group counseling or if the youth is better suited for individual counseling or some other form of support or intervention (Cooley, 2009). If the youth is presenting with severe mental health needs or has social challenges that prevent active participation with others, other forms of treatment will likely be more appropriate. Students who present themselves as monopolizing, dominating, or derogatory toward others may also not be good candidates for group work (Cooley, 2009; Yalom & Leszcz, 2005).

Group Size. Group size can vary depending on the content to be covered in the group, the age of the group members, and the severity of member's symptoms. It is generally recommended that most therapeutic groups contain five to eight members, though the practitioner should use discretion as to what is therapeutically indicated for the particular group (Haen & Aronson, 2016; Yalom & Leszcz, 2005).

Occurrence and Length

Group interventions with both short sessions and short overall time course have been supported in the literature (Gerrity & Delucia-Waack, 2006). Kulic and colleagues (2004) in their review of almost 100 published research studies on child and adolescent therapeutic group treatments found that over half of the groups ran a length of three months or less. Time-limited interventions are well supported in the school setting due to time constraints of the school day and academic year, as well as the amount of youth needing service. Though there is some variation, the preferred frequency for time-limited group therapy is not more than two sessions per week, with as few as six sessions total, or as many as 12, depending on the purpose and goals of the group (Center for Substance Abuse Treatment, 1999; Gerrity & Delucia-Waack, 2006). With regard to session length, it is recommended that children six years and under meet only for 20–30 minutes, children 6–9 years meet for 30–40 minutes, and children 9 years and older meet for no more than 75 minutes (Gerrity & Delucia-Waack, 2006). The group leader will need to adjust the amount of content covered in the group based on that group's specific make-up.

Developmental Considerations

No matter what intervention is chosen, it is imperative that it be adapted to the youth's developmental and cognitive level. Just because the group is marketed for a specific age range, the individual make-up of the group must be considered, and necessary adjustments made, such as modifying session content. The concept of mindfulness can be difficult to grasp, especially for young children, as they are often between the preoperational (2–7 years of age) and concrete operational stages (7–11 years of age), according to Jean Piaget's cognitive developmental theory, when abstract reasoning has not yet been developed (Piaget, 1969). Therefore, the use of objects, activities, and visuals that engage the young child's senses can be helpful in creating interest in and understanding of mindfulness concepts. The group curriculum overviewed in this chapter contains modifications based on age of the participants; however, it is essential that group leaders understand the specific members in their groups. Ideas for further adaptation are offered in Chapter 7 for children with developmental disabilities or social challenges or for those of varying cultural backgrounds.

Sample Group Curriculum

The curriculum outlined in this chapter is an example of a school-based group (grades 1–12) centered on mindfulness and ACT practices. This group was developed following the ACT model, with emphasis on mindfulness techniques. After development of this curriculum, we took this format and presented it to several school districts and at a state-wide conference (the California Association of School Psychologists (CASP)). Many of the activities included in the group sessions were run with the various participants (all school-related mental health professionals), as if they were group members. We did this to model for the participants how to run the sessions and activities, and to gain feedback from the group on the curriculum. Feedback forms were completed, with participants giving comments on each session and suggestions for improvement. These comments were then incorporated into completing the final draft of the curriculum, with several participants noting that they have since successfully run the group with youth at their schools.

Various adaptations based on age are offered throughout. Consistent with best practices for time-limited school-based groups, the curriculum is eight weeks in length, meeting once a week, for about 45–50 minutes each session, though the sessions can be further broken down and spaced more frequently, depending on the age of the children in the group and logistical constraints. The content of the group builds upon itself, both within each session, and across the span of the entire curriculum. In the first half of the curriculum, the focus is on forming group cohesion, educating group members on the stress response, and offering practical concrete tools for how to ground themselves via mindfulness. The latter sessions focus more on cognitive and acceptance techniques and tools, along with goal setting and relapse prevention.

As noted, we recommend the size of the group range between five to eight students, depending on age, developmental considerations, and presenting concern. As with any group, rapport building is critical; creating a safe setting will be of the utmost importance. Each session will have a similar format:

A brief initial mindfulness activity,
A discussion of the home practice,
An activity based on the topic for that session,
A home practice assignment,
A closing mindfulness activity.

Group Curriculum Outline

Session 1: Introduction to Mindfulness Practices

Objectives: Forming cohesion in the group, overviewing group ground rules, introducing mindfulness practices (ice breaker, group rules, 4x8 breaths)

Session 2: The Trouble with Thoughts

Objectives: Educating members on the role of the thinking mind in well-being. (brain structure, monkey mind, thought jar)

Session 3: Mindful Senses

Objectives: Introducing mindfulness techniques via the use of the senses. (5 senses technique, mindful eating)

Session 4: Thoughts, Revisited

Objectives: Introducing the idea of identifying negative, exclamatory thoughts and working with those. (Changing the Voice, Milk Technique)

Session 5: Acceptance and Mindfulness

Objectives: To learn about mindfulness through acceptance techniques. (the Clipboard Technique and the Chinese Finger Trap)

Session 6: Values and Goal Setting

Objectives: To goal set by identifying values and setting short- to long-term goals. (80th Birthday Party, Values List, Road to Success Diagram)

Session 7: When Roadblocks Happen

Objectives: Relapse prevention by returning to mindful breath and acceptance practices. Mountain Metaphor, Swamp Metaphor, Passengers on the Bus)

Session 8: Wrapping Up

Objectives: Review of curriculum, celebration of successes.

Ready, Set, Go!

To get started running this group in the schools, create buy-in from your referral sources – administration, teachers, and parents. Chapter 7 overviews best practices for creating engagement and buy-in. For example, attending a teachers' meeting to present the research-backed benefits of group therapy and to discuss the specific content to be covered in this group curriculum can assist with increasing buy-in. A letter to teachers soliciting student referrals (Form 5.1) and the Teacher Referral Form (Form 5.2) can assist with the referral process. Once you have identified possible group members, the Parent/Guardian Permission Letter (Form 5.3) can be sent to families of youth slated for inclusion. After the signed permissions have been received, screen each potential group member with a brief individual interview, as discussed earlier in this chapter. A Ready-Set-Go! Checklist (Form 5.4) is offered to keep track of the recommended steps for organizing a successful group.

Each session lists the physical materials needed for the session, a description of the activities to be conducted during that session, developmental adaptations, and ideas for debriefing activities. Review these areas before each session. The sessions can be broken down further, if necessary, depending on the specifics of the group you are running (developmental level, time allotted for each session, etc.). A suggestion for home practice is offered at the end of each session. Practitioner scripts and prompts are included, where appropriate. Though this group is suited for implementation within the school setting, the curriculum can also be easily adapted for private practice or clinic setting use.

Session 1: Introduction to Mindfulness Practices

Objectives:

- Rapport building
- Establish group guidelines
- Introduce mindfulness practices

Session Materials Needed:

- Large name tag stickers
- Pens
- Poster board or paper
- Optional: Bubbles, pinwheels (see developmental adaptations)

Total time: 45–50 minutes

Opening Statement:

PRACTITIONER: *Welcome to the group! We will be meeting once a week for the next eight weeks. As you know, the focus of our time together will be working on ways of helping our minds and bodies feel healthy. Let's start off by getting to know one another a bit.*

OPENING ACTIVITY: NAME TAG ART (10 MINUTES)

Materials:

- Large name tag stickers
- Colorful ink pens

Description:

Youth create name tags to wear during the first session. Tags are to contain both the youth's name and a word or drawing of one thing they like to do in their free time. Examples can be given (e.g., "My name is Melissa and I enjoy snowboarding, so I will draw a mountain with snow on it under my name."). It is helpful if the practitioner also creates a name tag to model for the youth the expectation of the activity.

Developmental Adaptations:

Children in younger grades or those with developmental delays may need assistance writing or drawing on their tags.

Activity Debrief:

Each group member will state their name and describe what activity they have written or drawn on their nametag.

After the name tag activity, transition to students sitting in a circle.

ESTABLISH GROUP GUIDELINES (10 MINUTES)

Materials:

- Either large poster board or writing paper
- Colorful ink pens

Description: Group guidelines and rules need to be established early to set the culture for future interactions. It is best to ask the group what rules they think would be helpful in establishing a trusting, respectful environment where everyone can feel heard. Following are examples of rules that you may want to include.

1. Listen while others are speaking.
2. Participate in group discussions and activities.
3. Use respectful language.
4. What is said in the group, stays in the group.

Developmental Adaptations:

Children in younger grades or those with developmental delays may benefit from the writing of the rules on a poster board that can be displayed at each group session. Older grades could benefit from a contract wherein group rules are agreed upon, listed, and signed by each member.

INTRODUCTION TO THE CONCEPT OF MINDFULNESS (15 MINUTES)

Materials:

* Optional: Bubbles, pinwheels (see developmental adaptations)

Description:

Start by asking the group members what they know about mindfulness. Have they ever heard of mindfulness? If so, what do they think it means? Next, define mindfulness and correct any misconceptions about it. Then, introduce 4x8 breathwork.

PRACTITIONER: *Have you ever heard the word "mindfulness" before?* (wait for responses). *Can anyone tell me what they think it means?* (listen and respond to responses). *Mindfulness is paying attention to the present moment without judging it in our thoughts. We will talk more about our thoughts in our next session. Today, we are going to talk about our breath and how the way we breathe can help us be right here, right now.*

Use seated posture (Form 3.3) with the youth seated in chairs. Demonstrate and explain the seated posture, discussing the idea of an erect spine and feet flat on the floor, with hands lying loosely in the lap. Practice 4x8 breathing with the group as outlined in the following script.

PRACTITIONER: *Today, we are going to try a type of breathing called 4 by 8 breathing. This means we are going to be taking deep breaths in to the count of 4, hold it briefly at the top, and let it out to the count of 8. In this way we are breathing out twice as long as we are breathing in. Let's all try it together.*

The children breathe in as the practitioner slowly counts *1-2-3-4,* pauses at the top, then counts slowly out *1-2-3-4-5-6-7-8.*

PRACTITIONER: *Good, let's do another. A deep breath in to the count of 4, and out to the count of 8* (practitioner continues this script, and models 4x8 breaths for another six to eight breaths).

PRACTITIONER: *And let's do one more together, briefly hold, and release your breath. Good.*

Developmental Adaptations:

For younger children or for those who are having a hard time producing smooth controlled in-breaths and out-breaths, the use of bubbles or pinwheels can be helpful. Deep in-breaths and elongated outbreaths are necessary for best effect when using each of these, i.e., more bubbles produced, longer pinwheel spins. A Hoberman sphere can also be used to help children practice breathing exercises, with the visual of each inhalation being coupled with the expansion of the sphere, and each exhalation paired with the contraction of the sphere. Metaphors, such as smelling a flower while taking a slow deep in-breath and blowing out a candle while exhaling, can also be used.

Activity Debrief:

Ask the group members what they noticed during the breathwork, and if they felt any differences after the breathwork compared to before. Ask if anyone noticed a greater awareness of what was around them after doing these kinds of breaths.

MINDFULNESS AS IT RELATES TO OUR LIVES (10 MINUTES)

Materials: None.

Description:

The goal of the following discussion is to help youth begin to see how mindfulness can be helpful in their lives. Discuss with group members the various scenarios below. Ask members if they have ever noticed these situations in their own lives.

Question Examples: *Have you ever:*

- *Had a hard time falling asleep because your mind has too many thoughts?*
- *Said something in the moment that you later wish you could take back?*
- *Felt angry and did something you later regretted?*
- *Been in a bad mood and you couldn't figure out why?*
- *Had a hard time focusing on something you are reading or working on?*
- *Felt nervous before a test or quiz?*
- *Walked to school or the park, then couldn't remember how you got there because you were so caught up in your thoughts?*
- *Not been able to stop thinking about something, even though the thing you are thinking about makes you feel anxious, mad, or sad?*

Developmental Adaptations:

The above questions can be altered, and the language adjusted based on age level. For example, for younger children, ask questions such as: *Have you ever felt mad and did something that got you in trouble?* or *Have you ever said something that hurt someone's feelings and you wished you had not said it?*

Activity Debrief:

Discuss with the youth that our thoughts can lead to feelings that are distracting and/or painful. These feelings can urge us to say and do things that we wish we had not. They can make it hard to focus and learn at times. Connect the idea that the more mindful we are, the more awareness we can have of our feelings and our behaviors, and what is around us. By increasing mindfulness, you are then better able to refrain from acting reactively to emotions or thoughts.

CLOSING ACTIVITY: HOME PRACTICE (5 MINUTES)

Encourage group members to take a few moments each day to practice the mindful breathing exercise taught in the session. Encourage them to use 4x8 breath in various situations and settings, such as before going to sleep, before taking a test, or on their way to school. They will have an opportunity to share their experiences in the next session. Thank the members for coming and sharing their time with one another.

Session 2: Mindful Senses

Objectives:
- Further rapport building
- Review of mindfulness and breathwork
- Helping members practice mindfulness through the five senses

Session Materials Needed:
- Foil wrapped chocolate candy or raisins

   Total time: 45–50 minutes

Opening Statement:

PRACTITIONER: *Today we will be focusing on the different ways we can practice being mindful. We will start, though, by getting to know one another a bit more through a short activity.*

OPENING ACTIVITY: A GREAT WIND BLOWS (10 MIN)

   Materials: A chair for each youth

   Description: This activity allows for movement and a way to have members learn more about one another and find common ground. Arrange chairs in a circle so that they all face the inside. Place one chair in the middle of the circle. With all the group members seated, the group leader sits in the chair in the middle to begin the game. Tell the members that they will be playing a game. The facilitator will call out a fact that other group members may share.

Those members who share that fact are to get up and move to another seat; if they do not share that fact, then the member stays seated. Let members know they will play a practice round to get the hang of it.

The group leader, who will begin as the caller, should call out "*A great wind blows for everyone who* _____." The blank should be filled in with such things as:

- ate cereal for breakfast
- has a younger sibling
- has swam in the ocean
- likes to play soccer
- enjoys camping
- plays video games

The members for whom this applies should stand up and change seats at least two chairs away from where they are currently sitting. If the fact applies to the caller, they will also get up and move to another seat in the circle. Whoever then winds up in the middle chair becomes the new caller. The group leader can continue to play, encouraging the new caller to complete the stem "*A great wind blows for everyone who* _____." If the leader does not continue to play, but instead assists another to be the caller e.g., make suggestions for what to say), one chair should be removed from the circle to ensure that one person always ends up as the caller. Tell members not to run or push into others to ensure safety.

Developmental Adaptations:

For younger children, the leader can always be the caller, coming up with the answers to the stem. Children simply move to a different seat if the answer pertains to them. For teens, encourage the answers to the stem to be more mature in nature (e.g., skis, has gone to the drive-in movies before, crams for finals, etc.).

Activity Debrief:

Discuss with the members how we may have more things in common with others than we realize. Encourage members to continue to find out more about one another as the weeks go on.

HOME PRACTICE REVIEW (5 MINUTES)

Talk with members about the 4x8 breathing exercise that was practiced during the last session. Discuss with members how these breaths can be used differently (e.g., to calm ourselves, to focus, to become more aware of what is around us, to help decrease our heart rate). Ask members for examples of how they used (or could have used) this exercise over the last week. Lead members in four 4x8 breaths (see Session 1).

ACTIVITY: 5 SENSES TECHNIQUE (15 MINUTES)

Materials: None

Description:

The 5 Senses Technique uses the youths' senses to help them be more aware of the present moment. The following script is an example of how to guide students through this activity.

Practitioner: (Start the discussion with a brief review of mindfulness (e.g., what it is, why it can be helpful). *Now we are going to use our five senses to help us to be right here in this moment. Can you tell me what the five senses are? Seeing is one.*

Wait for responses, filling in the others (hearing, tasting, touching, smelling) if missed by the group members.

That's right, those are all of our senses. Thinking is not a sense, but sometimes we think about things so much that we miss what is actually happening around us. Often the way to really know what is actually happening is by using our five senses.

We will start by taking in a few deep breaths, as we have been working on. Take in a deep breath in through your nose to the count of four, hold it briefly, then out to the count of eight. Good, let's do another.

Model for the youth taking in these deep breaths. Take four deep breaths with them.

Good, now, either soften your eyes, without focusing hard on any one thing, and look toward the floor or, if you are comfortable, close your eyes.

Model this for the members.

As we continue to take in those deep 4 by 8 breaths, we will turn our attention to just what we are hearing right now in the room.

Here note for the members what sounds are being heard either in or outside the room. Modify the following sample to match what is being heard in that moment.

Perhaps you hear the sound of the air conditioner, or the clock ticking. You may hear sounds outside the room, like people talking or traffic going by. Just focus on your deep breaths, and what you are hearing right now.

Good, now notice the weight of your body in your chair. Notice the solidness of the floor underneath your feet. Note the temperature of the air on your face and hands. Just be right here. Notice the parts of your back that are touching the chair and the parts of your back that are not, and the difference between those. We will continue to take our deep breaths in to the count of four, and out to the count of eight.

Notice if you have any taste on your tongue. Note if you can smell any smells or scents in the room.

Now open your eyes and look around the room. You may notice that colors seem brighter, and lines on objects are sharper and clearer. Perhaps you notice something in the room that you had not noticed before.

Good, and we will take in one last deep breath, and let it out.

Developmental Adaptations:

This activity can be broken down for younger children, with just one sense at a time being practiced and then briefly discussed before moving on to the next sense. The cadence of the breaths can also be altered so that they are not so elongated for young children, for example, 2x4.

Activity Debrief:

Ask the members how that exercise was for them. Have them describe what it was like to use their five senses in this way. Ask if they noticed anything in the room they had not noticed earlier, such as when they came into the group that day.

ACTIVITY: MINDFUL EATING (10 MINUTES)

Materials:

• Foil wrapped chocolate candies, raisins, or another small snack item (at least 1 per member)

Description:

In this activity, youth will practice mindful eating through use of all of their senses. The following script uses chocolate but can be adapted for other small snack items.

Each group member will be given a piece of foil wrapped chocolate, such as a Hershey's Kiss. Tell the youth not to eat the chocolate, but instead to hold the chocolate in their hands.

Practitioner: *While holding the chocolate in your hand, we are going to pretend like we are visitors from another planet and are experiencing this new food for the first time. We are going to use all of our five senses to investigate this object.*

Model holding the chocolate between your index finger and thumb, bringing it up to your face.

Look at the object as you hold it in your fingers. Notice what it looks like. Is it shiny or dull, bumpy or smooth? What color is it? Does the light catch the object on some areas differently than others? What does the weight of the object feel like in your hand?

Next, we are going to use our sense of hearing to listen. Can we hear any sounds as we unwrap our objects?

Slowly unwrap your object, modeling for the youth your intense focus on the process.

Now we are going to use our sense of smell to smell the object. Breathe deeply as you hold your object under your nose. Notice if you can smell any scents as you breathe in deeply. Good, let's try that again.

Model breathing in deeply as you hold the chocolate under your nose.

Now, place the object on your tongue and just hold it there. What does it feel like? Can you taste anything? Now slowly chew your object, starting with just one bite. Does the object change form as you bite it? Is there more flavor now that you can taste?

Pause a moment while the youth chew the object.

Good, now, as you swallow the object, do you notice any taste left on your tongue?

Developmental Adaptations:

Most ages can participate without variation.

Activity Debrief:

Engage the youth in a discussion about the exercise. Ask how this was different from how they usually eat a piece of candy. What did they notice as they were engaged in this activity? How did eating mindfully feel different than if they had eaten the chocolate more quickly? Did they feel more or less satisfied? Did they enjoy it more or less?

CLOSING ACTIVITY: HOME PRACTICE

Encourage group members to use their five senses mindfully when taking first bites of their next meals.

Session 3: The Trouble with Thoughts

Objectives:

* Further rapport building
* Review of mindfulness and breathwork
* Educating members on thoughts as related to the nervous system

Session Materials Needed:

- Brain Structure Handout (5.1)
- Sunglasses (1 per member, different shaded lenses, if possible)
- Small plastic jars
- Glycerin or corn syrup
- Glitter of various colors
- Jug of water

Total time: 45–50 minutes

Opening Statement:

PRACTITIONER: *Today we will be focusing on mindfulness and our thoughts. After we talk about how our mindful eating went over the last week, we will start with a short activity to better understand how our thoughts can color the way we see things and how we respond.*

HOME PRACTICE REVIEW (5 MINUTES)

Encourage group members to share their experiences of eating mindfully over the last week. If members forgot to do this, discuss the mindful eating activity practiced last week and how they can apply those skills using their five senses to their next meal.

OPENING ACTIVITY: OUR BRAINS ON THOUGHTS OVERVIEW (20 MINUTES)

Materials:

- Brain structure handout
- Sunglasses (different shades/colored lenses if possible)

Description:

Discuss with the members how mindfulness, focusing on the present moment without judging it, can help us in different ways. The following script can be adapted for this discussion:

PRACTITIONER: *Mindfulness is about paying attention to what is happening in this moment. Often our thoughts take us out of the present moment. We may find we are thinking about things that happened in the past, or about things that may happen in the future. When this happens, we are not paying attention to what is happening in the present anymore.*
    Pass out Brain Structure Handout 5.1.
PRACTITIONER: *Our brains are wired to react in stressful situations. They automatically prepare us to respond by either fighting, fleeing, or freezing. This*

is helpful if we need to protect ourselves from a bear or tiger. The part of the brain that helps us to react this way is called the amygdala.

Point to this area on the handout.

PRACTITIONER: *When we are stressed, the amygdala sends messages to get our bodies and minds ready to fight or run away from the danger. Other parts of our brain shut down during this time. These parts are called our hippocampus, also known as our memory house, and our prefrontal cortex, which is really important for making good decisions and planning.*

Point to the hippocampus and the prefrontal cortex.

PRACTITIONER: *Out of the areas I just pointed to, which two do you think would be most important during, say, a math test or while we are in a class discussion?*

Wait for responses; discuss how the prefrontal cortex and the hippocampus are very important to make good choices, think things through, and remember things.

PRACTITIONER: *That's right, the prefrontal cortex and the hippocampus are really important when at school. In danger, our amygdala's job is to make us act fast without spending time thinking or weighing our choices. Our heart rate starts to speed up and we may start breathing faster. This gets our bodies ready to run quickly or fight the threat. This is good if we are in danger, like if a tiger jumps out at us, but not so good if we are taking a math test.*

The problem is our thoughts can often act like tigers. Some thoughts can trigger the same reactions in our bodies as if a real danger were in front of us.

Mindfulness can help us slow things down in two ways. The first is through our breath. Slowing down our breath slows our heart rate and calms us. Second, mindfulness helps us to see our thoughts more clearly. It can help us see that thoughts sometimes trick us. Mindfulness can help us stay calm and in control when our thoughts are triggering a false emergency.

Ask the group members to raise their hands if they have ever had the following thoughts:

- That person must be mad at me because they didn't smile or say "hi" when I walked up.
- I know I didn't study enough for my test; I am going to fail.
- I feel like something bad is going to happen today.
- I am so overwhelmed with all I have to do.

Discuss with the members how these kinds of thoughts can color our experiences of ourselves, others, and the world around us. Bring out the different colored sunglasses and talk with members about how thoughts can change the way things look to us. Have members try on the different glasses and discuss how the room looks different with the different shades of the lenses.

PRACTITIONER: *Do you notice how the room gets darker with some of the lenses? Now imagine that you wake up in the morning and have the thought, "This is going to be a terrible day." How do you imagine things might look? How differently would you feel about your morning when having that thought? Just like putting on a pair of sunglasses, our thoughts can color how we see things.*

Mindfulness helps us notice that we are having thoughts, and that we can notice them without having them color our experiences inside and outside. It's kind of like this, (demonstrate putting on the glasses, and saying), *"It is going to be a terrible day."* (Then take off the glasses, and say), *"I am having the thought that it will be a terrible day. It is just a thought, not a fact. I can choose to notice this thought without having it change the way things look and feel to me."*

Developmental Adaptations:

For younger children, the discussion about the brain structure can be taken out, focusing instead on how the different sunglasses make the room look different, and how our thoughts can do that too. Share some examples of thoughts, such as, *"My teacher is mad at me," "I am stupid," "My friend doesn't like me."* Discuss how these thoughts can make things look and feel different, and that they are just thoughts and may not really be how things are.

Activity Debrief:

Encourage the group members to share different thoughts that they have had that may have "shaded" their day in a certain way. Talk about these thoughts in relation to the sunglasses. Discuss how some thoughts can be so troublesome that they take us out of using our hippocampus and our prefrontal cortex. This makes it hard to think clearly, plan, or remember things. Discuss how thoughts are not facts; just because we think it, doesn't mean it's true.

THOUGHT JAR ACTIVITY (20 MINUTES)

Materials:

- Clear glass or plastic jars
- Glitter of various colors
- Water
- Glycerin

Description:

Place the jars and the containers of glitter out on a table and have the members gather around. Instruct youth to put glitter of their choosing in their jars, letting them know that the glitter is going to represent different kinds of thoughts that we have. Once they have sprinkled glitter into their jars, fill the youth's jars with water, dropping in a few drops of glycerin, and leaving a little air at the top. Screw the lids on tightly.

PRACTITIONER: *Now that you have glitter and water in your jar, go ahead and give it a few good shakes. See how the glitter is swirling around in your jars. This is like how our minds become when we are absorbed in our thinking minds. The glitter is like our thoughts, all jumbled and scattered in our minds. If we stop and become quiet, we can settle our minds. Notice that the glitter settles to the bottom of the jar when we stop shaking it up. We haven't deleted the thoughts, but instead have allowed them to settle. Your thoughts are still there, as the glitter is still there. When we allow the jar to sit without shaking it, the glitter settles to the bottom and the water is clear. When we become quiet and mindful, our thoughts are not stirred up and our minds become clear.*

Developmental Adaptations:

You may adjust the language used in the previous script if deemed too advanced for some students. For example, focus on shaking the jar, then stopping and allowing the glitter to settle, stating, "*This is like when we have thoughts. Our minds start swirling, just like the glitter in our jars. When we stop and take a few deep breaths, it can help us to feel calmer.*"

Activity Debrief:

Ask the youth for examples of times when they have noticed their thoughts swirling like glitter in the jars. Discuss how our minds can become clearer when we become mindful and are simply aware of our thoughts, instead of continuing to shake them up.

CLOSING ACTIVITY: HOME PRACTICE (5 MINUTES)

Instruct the youth to shake up their jars and then hold them still. Then, while remaining still, ask them to take in four 4x8 breaths. Highlight that they can use deep breathing to calm their minds and bodies, just as the glitter has become still in their jars. Encourage members to refer to their jars over the next week to remind them to practice this mindfulness exercise. Let them know they can share their experiences of using their 4x8 breaths to help settle their thoughts in the next session.

Session 4: Thoughts Revisited

Objectives:

- To review mindfulness work
- To introduce the idea of cognitive defusion
- To introduce the idea of the "puppy mind"

Session Materials Needed:

- Sticky notes (e.g., Post-its)
- Optional: *The Puppy Mind* by Nance (2016)

Total time: 45–50 minutes

Opening Statement:

PRACTITIONER: *Today, we are going to focus more on our thoughts, and how we can help to settle our thoughts more easily, or at least change how they can "shade" our lives, like the sunglasses last week. First, we are going to talk about your home practice and complete a mindfulness breathing exercise.*

HOME PRACTICE REVIEW (5 MINUTES)

Discuss with the youth how their experiences were with their thought jars over the last week. Leave time for youth to share if they shook up their jars coupled with their breathwork, as discussed in the last session (e.g., before bedtime, before going to school, etc.). Encourage the youth to continue using their glitter jars and 4x8 breathing at various times and in various situations over the coming week to continue their mastery of this mindfulness practice.

Identify one thought that each youth has had over the last week that has "jumped out" at them like a tiger, as discussed in the last session. Have the youth write down a word or thought that has been upsetting to them over the last week on a sticky note (help younger children or those who need assistance by writing it down for them). Discuss with the youth how these words or thoughts that we repeat to ourselves are often very "sticky," just like the note itself. Have the youth set aside the note to be used later in the session. Let youth know they do not have to share what their thought is with the rest of the group. The group leader should also write down a thought (e.g., "I blew it," or "I will never get this right") in order to use this as an example later in the session.

OPENING ACTIVITY: BREATHING MEDITATION (15 MINUTES)

Materials: None
Description:
This activity will help youth to focus on their breathing and increase awareness of their thoughts without becoming absorbed by them.

PRACTITIONER: *We are going to continue our 4x8 breaths today and notice what thoughts come up as we breathe. Ready? Let's take in a deep breath to the count of four, briefly hold it, then let it out to the count of eight.*
    Continue to take in six more 4x8 breaths with the youth, guiding them through each breath via counting.
PRACTITIONER: *Now, close your eyes, if you feel comfortable, or lower your gaze. We are going to continue to put our attention on our deep 4x8 breaths and just be here in the room together. Thoughts may come into our minds as we are breathing. When a thought comes into your mind, imagine putting it in a bubble, like in a cartoon when the characters have thoughts in bubbles above their heads. Then watch the thought float away in the bubble. Let's try that. Notice the thought you are having, place it in a bubble, and watch the thought float away. Then come back to your breathing.*
    Continue to take in deep breaths to the count of four and let them out to the count of eight. When you notice the next thought come into your mind, place that thought in another bubble, and watch it float away, bringing your awareness back to your deep breathing.

Developmental Adaptations:

Imagery may not be as effective with particularly young children or those with cognitive delays, as abstract thinking is more challenging. In this case, attention can be placed more on the mindfulness and body scan techniques, as demonstrated next. Alternatively, actual bubbles could be used wherein children breathe in deeply, then breathe a slow outbreath, as they imagine their thoughts inserted into the actual bubbles blown by the group leader as they float away.

Activity Debrief:

Discuss with youth how we can alter the power our thoughts have over our moods and experiences. The more we notice our thoughts without having them shade our experiences, as in the sunglasses activity, the more mindful we can be. With increased mindfulness, we are able to make purposeful choices about how we interact with our thoughts and experiences – holding onto those thoughts and experiences that bring us calmness or joy, while letting go of those that don't.

ALTERNATIVE ACTIVITY

BODY SCAN SCRIPT

Encourage the group members to get comfortable and settle into their chairs. Prompt them to begin engaging in some 4x8 breaths and then move them through the following exercise.

Today, we are going to do a quick body scan. This involves focusing our attention on any sensations we might be having in our bodies. We aren't trying to change these sensations, just notice them.

Breath: *First, let's turn our attention to our breath. Continue taking some 4x8 breaths. As you do, see if you can notice what the air feels like as you first breathe in. Is the air cold or warm as it enters your mouth or nose? See if you can follow your breath from the moment it enters your mouth or nose, until it enters your lungs. Notice how your body feels different as the air enters your lungs. Finally, follow your breath as it exits your body. Has the temperature of the air changed? Does your body feel any different?*

Feet: *Next, I want you to turn your attention to your feet. See if you can notice how your feet feel as they make contact with the floor. Do your feet feel warm or cold, tense, or relaxed? Take a moment to just notice your feet. And if your attention starts to drift to other thoughts, just notice that, and bring your attention back to your feet.*

Legs: *Now let's focus our attention on our legs. See if you can notice how it feels for your clothes to make contact with your legs. Are your legs feeling calm or do they want to move? Are they feeling heavy or light? Just take a moment to notice any sensations in your legs.*

Stomach: *Okay, now let's pay attention to our tummies. Notice how your tummy changes as you breathe in and out. See if you can identify any other sensations your tummy might be feeling. Are you full or hungry? Can you feel your shirt making contact with your tummy? Spend a few moments just noticing any sensations happening in your tummy. And if you notice that your mind has wandered off, gently bring your focus back to your tummy.*

Hands: *Good, now we are going to shift our focus to our hands. Notice where your hands are currently located. Are they in your lap, holding onto the chair, or clasped together? Are they feeling cold or warm; tense or relaxed? No need to move them or do anything with them. Just take a moment to notice them.*

Arms: *Next, we are going to pay attention to our arms. Try tuning your attention into noticing what your arms are coming into contact with. Are your* *arms feeling heavy or light? Do you notice any tingling, goosebumps, or other sensations?*

Chest: *Now, shift your focus to your chest. See if you can focus your mind on simply following the rise and fall of your chest as you continue to breathe in and out. Follow this rise and fall for several breaths. If you notice your mind has been wandering, simply bring your attention back to noticing the rise and fall of your chest.*

Shoulders: *Let's pay attention to our shoulders now. Notice the positioning of your shoulders. Are they tense or loose; are they raised or relaxed? Spend a few moments just focused on noticing any sensations in your shoulders.*

Face: *Finally, center your focus on your face and head. What type of expression do you have on your face right now? As you notice your face, notice if you feel any desire to change your facial expression. If your facial expression has changed since paying attention to your facial muscles, notice any changes to how your face feels.*

End by taking a few final 4x8 breaths.

Alternative Activity Debrief: Discuss with the youth how paying more attention to our bodies can help us become more aware of our internal experiences. Note that while many youth find a body scan relaxing, that is not the goal. Instead, the goal is to increase present-moment awareness, and ultimately, acceptance of these experiences.

ACTIVITY: CHANGING THE VOICE (10 MINUTES)

Materials: None

Description:

When we have a thought that is negative it can often be experienced as a threat; thoughts can jump out at us like bears or tigers in our minds. Often, we hear these painful, repetitive thoughts in an authoritative tone. These negative thoughts can significantly taint how you experience the present moment. They can cause emotional reactions and behaviors that do not match what is actually happening in the present. Changing the tone of the internal thought can create more flexibility in thinking (Harris, 2009).

PRACTITIONER: *Today, we are going to take the thought that you wrote down on your sticky note and play with it a little bit. Tell me this, when you have this thought, is it said, "in a very important voice, like this" (practitioner says this in a deep, authoritative tone) so you really feel you must listen to it?*

Wait for youth to respond, being certain that they understand what you mean.

PRACTITIONER: *Yes, often when we say negative things to ourselves it is said in an "important voice" tone, which makes us pay attention to it and believe it. Now tell me this, what would happen if we changed the tone of the voice for this thought. What if, instead of the "very important voice tone"* (practitioner uses deep voice again here*), the tone of the voice was silly, say, that of Mickey Mouse's voice?*

Pause here, then give an example of a thought you wrote down on your sticky note as outlined next.

PRACTITIONER: *Instead of the important voice of "I will never get this right"* (uses deep voice, reading their own note*), instead use a Mickey Mouse voice like, "I will never get this right"* (practitioner uses exaggerated, high pitched silly voice).

Group members likely will have some response here, often laughing.

PRACTITIONER: *Yes, that's right. It is really hard to pay serious attention to a Mickey Mouse voice. This helps us see that it is just a thought we are having, not a fact, not a real story of how things actually are.*

Developmental Adaptations:

For younger children (e.g., grades first to third) read the book *Puppy Mind* by Nance (2016). Discuss the book after, asking the youth ways that they can be kind and peaceful with their "puppy minds."

Activity Debrief:

Discuss how thoughts are just thoughts, and sometimes they are not helpful to us. These can also be called "garbage thoughts." When we begin to see that thoughts are not necessarily how things really are, we can begin to have more control over our experiences.

ACTIVITY: MILK TECHNIQUE (5 MINUTES)

Materials: None

Description:

A defusion technique popular with youth is the milk exercise. It was first used in the early 1900s by Tichener (1916) to decrease the power that certain words hold.

PRACTITIONER: *We've been talking a lot about how sad you feel when certain negative thoughts, or garbage thoughts, come into your head, like "I'm stupid," right? I want to do an exercise with you all today that can help you in moments when you're having mean thoughts like that about yourselves. First,*

I want you to think of the word "milk." When you hear that word, what comes to mind? I want you to list out anything that you can think of – other words, images, memories, and so on.

Allow group members time to respond.

PRACTITIONER: *Great! Really nice job! Okay, now I want you to do something else. It may seem kind of goofy. I want you to repeat the word "milk" out loud over and over again until I tell you to stop.*

Have the group members continue to repeat the word for 60 seconds.

PRACTITIONER: *Nice work! What did you notice about the word "milk" as you kept saying it over and over again?* Give members time to respond, then proceed. *Yes, at first, it may have just felt like you were saying the word "milk" but then after you kept saying it, the sounds all may have started to run together. Maybe it didn't even feel like you were saying a real word anymore! Okay, now I want to try it with another word that might have more difficult emotions and memories attached to it. Let's try now by saying the word "stupid" over and over again.*

> **Developmental Adaptations:** The debrief may be simplified, perhaps using actual sticky notes that would become less sticky if attached and detached to a wall or our foreheads over and over again (see the following).

Activity Debrief:

Discuss with the youth their experience of this activity. Ask about how the word may have changed over time as they continued to repeat it. Discuss how often people find that words repeated again and again lose their meaning. Refer the youth back to the words on their sticky notes. Discuss how this technique could be used with those words. It might help the youth see that words are just sounds and that they do not need to hold power over us. Repetition can reduce their "stickiness," just like the sticky notes would become less sticky if attached and detached to a wall or our foreheads over and over again.

CLOSING ACTIVITY: HOME PRACTICE

Over the next week, encourage the youth to catch themselves having the thoughts that they wrote down on their sticky notes. When they catch them, repeat the thought in a Mickey Mouse voice in their heads. Tell them to remind themselves it is just a thought they are having. Then come back to the present moment. Suggest that they also use the "milk technique" and their deep breathing to help reduce the "stickiness" of these thoughts.

Session 5: Acceptance and Mindfulness

Objectives:

- To overview breathing and defusion techniques
- To introduce the tenants of acceptance
- To couple acceptance and breathwork

Session Materials Needed:

- A clipboard
- A blank piece of paper (one for each member)
- Chinese finger traps (one for each member)
- Optional: *What Does It Mean to be Present?* by DiOrio (2010)

Opening Statement:

PRACTITIONER: *Today, we are going to focus on how to use our breath and our relationship to our thoughts to feel as healthy as we can, both physically and emotionally. We will review our home practice activity, then start with a breathing exercise.*

HOME PRACTICE REVIEW (5 MINUTES)

Discuss with the youth if they noticed any "sticky" thoughts over the last week. Ask them about their use of the "Mickey Mouse" voice or the "milk technique," or if they were able to remind themselves that the thoughts they had were just thoughts. Encourage youth to continue to use these techniques when "sticky" thoughts arise.

OPENING ACTIVITY: MANTRAS (10 MINUTES)

Materials: None

Description:

Mantras are sayings that can be repeated internally or out loud as a form of focused meditation. It allows our thoughts to become focused and shifted away from other less helpful and/or negative thoughts. The following meditation introduces the use of mantras with group members.

PRACTITIONER: *Today, we are going to talk about mantras. A mantra is something that we can say to ourselves inside of our heads or out loud. It can help us in different ways, such as to feel calmer and more supported. I will now show you some of these mantras as I do some 4x8 breaths* (as the group leader breathes in, the leader will repeat the beginning of the mantra, then, while breathing out, will repeat the end of the mantra).

Breathing in I am calm (practitioner breathes in to the count of 4), *breathing out I am relaxed* (practitioner breathes out to the count of 8).

Breathing in I am safe (practitioner breathes in), *breathing out my needs are met* (practitioner breathes out).

Breathing in I am loved (practitioner breathes in), *breathing out I am cared for* (practitioner breathes out).

Repeat the above mantras aloud as you instruct the group members to breathe in to the count of 4, and out to the count of 8. Do 2 rounds of the above mantras with the youth.

Next, encourage the youth to select a mantra that resonates with them. Provide some examples, such as 'I am enough.' or 'I believe in myself." or 'I've got this." Instruct the group members to breathe in to the count of 4, and out to the count of 8, as they internally recite their personally chosen mantras. Do 2 additional rounds of this with the youth.

Developmental Adaptations:

For younger children, simplify the mantra to a single word (e.g., calm, relaxed, enough) that is repeated as they practice their breathwork.

Activity Debrief:

Ask the youth to share their experiences with this exercise. If youth feel comfortable, they are welcome to share the personal mantra they selected with the other group members. Sometimes it can be helpful for youth to write down their mantra so they can remember it for future practice. They might carry it with them or post it somewhere noticeable, for example, on the back of their bedroom door, taped inside their school binder, and so on.

ACTIVITY: CLIPBOARD TECHNIQUE (15 MINUTES)

Materials:

* Clipboard or another flat thin object
* Blank paper, one page for each member

Description:

There are many variations on this technique, though typically it involves the practitioner using a solid object, such as a clipboard, as a metaphor for the thoughts, feelings, behaviors, or situations with which the youth is struggling (Harris, 2009). The practitioner instructs the youth to do various things with the object to illustrate how they struggle with these challenges. The youth being "flooded" by the challenge and trying to push away or distract themselves from the challenge are acted out. Acceptance of the challenge is then also acted out. Following is a script for this technique.

PRACTITIONER: Pass out one sheet of blank paper to each member. *Today, we are going to do something a little different with the negative thoughts that you have been having. We will begin by writing down a thought that has been hard for you on this blank paper. It could be the same thought you wrote down last week on your sticky notes, or it could be a different thought. You do not have to share what you write down with anyone else.*

    Practitioner picks up the clipboard. *Could I get one volunteer to start this activity?* Wait for a volunteer or choose a group member to start. *OK, I want you to imagine that this clipboard I am holding represents a difficult thought that you are having. I would like you to take it in your hands and grip it as tightly as you can so that I won't be able to pull it away from you.*

    Practitioner hands the clipboard to the volunteer youth, modeling the gripping action if the youth is unclear as to what to do.

    Good, now I would like you to hold the clipboard up in front of your face to where you can't see me anymore. Bring it up close to your face to where it is almost touching your nose. Good. Now, how easy do you think it would be to continue to have a conversation with me while you are holding your thought so tightly?

    Wait for youth to respond. If youth doesn't respond or says "I don't know" suggest the following.

PRACTITIONER: *Do you imagine over time you might start to feel distracted or tired gripping that so tightly?*

    Wait for youth to respond, then continue.

PRACTITIONER: *And what is your view of the room while you are holding onto this so tight?*

    Youth should respond along the lines of it being hard to see you or anything around them.

PRACTITIONER: *Yes, it is hard to be so absorbed in this thought and still be able to see clearly what is going on around you. How easy would it be to do the things that you enjoy doing, like drawing, petting a dog, or watching TV right now?* If possible, fill in activities that are pleasurable for the youth here.

    Youth should respond along the lines that it would be difficult, if not impossible.

PRACTITIONER: *Yeah, when we are all caught up in difficult thoughts, it can be almost impossible to see or do anything else. OK, you can release the clipboard now.*

Youth hands clipboard back to practitioner.

PRACTITIONER: *Would it be OK if we tried something else with the clipboard? Can I have another volunteer?*

Be sure to sit or stand next to the volunteer member, so you each can have contact with the clipboard.

PRACTITIONER: *The clipboard still represents the thought you have been struggling with. What I would like for you to do now is place both of your hands flat on the clipboard here, and I am going to place my hands on the other side. Now push the clipboard away from you. Push it firmly, but not so hard as to knock me over!*

As the youth pushes, the practitioner pushes back to match their intensity.

PRACTITIONER: *Good, keep pushing. You don't like this thought. You want to get rid of it, to make it go away. So, here you are, trying hard to push this stuff away. But do you notice it's not going anywhere? How easy would it be to continue to have a conversation with me for the rest of our meeting time together as you are pushing like this?*

Wait for youth to respond.

PRACTITIONER: *I would imagine it would get tiring and distracting. How easy would it be for you to do the things you enjoy doing, such as drawing, petting a dog, or watching TV?* Fill in activities that are pleasurable for the youth here, if possible.

Youth should respond it would not be possible or very difficult.

PRACTITIONER: *OK, good. Now go ahead and set the clipboard in your lap. The clipboard still represents the thought that is hard for you. Do you notice that it is still there?*

Youth should respond that they do notice it.

PRACTITIONER: *Sure, you notice it is still there, but I am guessing there is a lot less effort and energy given to it. How easy would it be now for us to continue to have our conversation?*

Youth should respond along the lines of it being easy or easier.

PRACTITIONER: *And how easy would it be for you to do the things you may enjoy doing, such as drawing, petting a dog, or watching TV?* (fill in activities that are pleasurable for the youth here, if possible).

Youth should respond that it would be easier.

PRACTITIONER: *So, no longer is it the only thing you can see* (practitioner holds an imaginary clipboard up in front of their face), *and no longer are you trying to get rid of this thought* (practitioner demonstrates the pushing motion). *Instead, you notice that it is still there, but you are devoting less energy toward it, just noticing it without attaching to it or it being so sticky. You can see things more clearly around you and you have more energy to do the things you love to do.*

Now each of you will pair up with the group member next to you. Try holding up your papers tightly in front of your faces; then switch to pushing the paper back and forth as we just did.

Allow time for members to do these actions. Have each pair of students designate who will hold the paper the first round and second round. After practicing once, instruct students to trade roles and repeat the activity so each student gets a turn holding their paper.

Good, now just lay the paper in your lap. You haven't gotten rid of your thought, but it's not flooding you, being the only thing you see. Instead of trying to push away and delete the thought, which we know can't happen, we are simply aware of the thought. We are not letting it take up so much of our awareness and energy.

Developmental Adaptations:

For children in middle elementary school or younger, an alternative activity to consider is reading *What Does It Mean to be Present?* by DiOrio (2010). Discuss the book with the members and ways that they can practice being present before the next session.

Activity Debrief:

Ask the youth to share what their experience was like in their pairs. What did they notice? Encourage the youth to consider this metaphor over the next week and to begin to change their relationship with their thoughts. In later sessions, the clipboard metaphor can be referred to when the practitioner notices that the youth is either feeling flooded by their thoughts, feelings, or memories, or trying to distract themselves or push away these experiences.

ACTIVITY: CHINESE FINGER TRAPS (5 MINUTES)

Materials:

- Chinese finger traps

Description:

Another common acceptance metaphor used in ACT is that of the Chinese finger trap (Hayes & Smith, 2005). In this technique, the practitioner discusses with the youth how, the more you struggle to get your fingers out of the trap, the greater its hold. However, once the struggle stops and you relax, the trap releases and your fingers can be freed.

Hand out the finger traps to each member, discussing how our thoughts can grip us just like the traps. The more we struggle, the more we are stuck. Then model for them relaxing your hands, taking in a few deep 4x8 breaths. Note how it can be easier to release the hold of the finger trap or thought when we become still and mindful.

Developmental Adaptations:

Consider simplifying the language used, if necessary.

Activity Debrief:

Discuss with the youth that the mind is also like the finger trap: the more we struggle with our thoughts, the greater their hold. However, we can use mindfulness and breathwork to more easily drop the struggle of our thinking minds.

CLOSING ACTIVITY: HOME PRACTICE

Suggest referencing the metaphor of the clipboard and the finger trap over the next week to help "release the grip" of the challenging thoughts the youth may be having. Encourage the use of mantras and deep breathing at bedtime, as well as during times when they are feeling stressed or experiencing strong emotions.

Session 6: Values and Goal Setting

Objectives:

- To identify values
- To aid in goal identification
- To help in short-term and long-term goal setting

Session Materials Needed:

- Values List Handout (5.2)
- Road Map to Success Handout (5.3)
- Ink Pens
- Optional Activity Materials:

  Leaves on a Stream Handout
  A big piece of butcher paper with a river pre-drawn or painted on it
  Pre-cut paper leaves
  Tape or glue sticks
  Scissors

Note: Though values and goal setting are often introduced early on in the ACT model, they are offered here in Session 6 instead as a way to generalize learned skills of mindfulness, acceptance, and defusion techniques and to support students in continuing to use these skills after completion of the group.

Opening Statement:

PRACTITIONER: *Today, we are going to focus on how we can identify what we value and care about in our lives. When we know what we value, we are better able to set goals we want to work toward.*

HOME PRACTICE REVIEW (5 MINUTES)

Review last week's material including mantras, the Clip Board, and the Finger Trap exercises. Were they able to continue these practices over the past week? Did they find these practices to be helpful? Anything that felt challenging for them in using these practices? Ask for specific examples from the youth of how they used these practices over the past week.

PRACTITIONER: *Now, let's try a mindfulness exercise that can help us continue to work on becoming less attached to our thoughts.*

OPENING ACTIVITY: LEAVES ON A STREAM MEDITATION (10 MIN.; ADAPTED FROM HARRIS, 2009)

Materials:

* None

Description:

The Leaves on a Stream meditation can help youth identify and defuse from thoughts, becoming less attached to them.

Begin with taking in four 4x8 breaths with the youth. Then proceed with the following script.

PRACTITIONER: *As you continue to take in your deep, four by eight breaths, I want you to imagine a beautiful, slow-moving stream. The water is flowing over rocks, around trees, and through a valley. Once in a while, a big leaf drops into the stream and floats away down the river. Imagine you are sitting beside the stream, watching the leaves float by.*

Now become conscious of your thoughts. Each time a thought pops into your mind, imagine that it is written on one of those leaves. If it is easier, imagine placing the words from your mind on the leaf. Stay as you are beside the stream and allow the leaves to keep flowing by. Don't try to make the stream go faster or slower, and don't try to change what thoughts are placed on the leaves.

If you notice you are mentally somewhere else, and the stream or leaves have disappeared, just notice that this has happened, and gently bring yourself back to the stream and notice your thoughts on the leaves.

Allow pauses in the script to allow time for the youth to imagine the stream without interruption. Small prompts, such as, "As you take in this next deep breath and let it out, notice the flow of the stream and the leaves holding your thoughts as they make their way along," can be offered to help the youth refocus and continue in the imagery. Allow three to four minutes of practice with this exercise, depending on the youth's ability to participate in this exercise.

Developmental Adaptations:

This activity may be too cognitively complex for younger children. For younger children, or youth who are more concrete or respond well to visuals, consider using the alternative Leaves on a Stream art activity described next.

Activity Debrief:

Encourage the youth to share their experiences. Was there anything challenging about this exercise? Did they lose track of the stream and began thinking about other things? Did their mind try to slow the stream down or make the leaves get stuck? Did they notice that and were they able to come back to the stream and leaves as they were intended? Continuing to practice this will allow the youth to have greater awareness of themselves when lost in thought and to be better able to return to the present.

ALTERNATIVE ACTIVITY: LEAVES ON A STREAM ART PROJECT (10 MINUTES)

Materials:

- A big piece of butcher paper with a river pre-drawn or painted on it
- Pre-cut paper leaves
- Small pieces of paper (smaller than the leaves, perhaps the size of a sticky note)
- Tape or glue sticks
- Scissors

Description:

Pass out small pieces of paper to the members. Tell the members to write a word or thought that bothers them on the paper, or they can draw a small picture representing the thought that troubles them, such as "unlikeable," "dumb," or any thought that is overly negative and upsetting.

Once the thought is written or drawn on the small piece of paper, have them cut the paper into small pieces so that the content is no longer recognizable. The members will then glue the small shreds of paper onto a pre-cut paper leaf like an abstract collage.

After the leaves have been decorated, have the members glue the leaves onto the butcher paper stream, as if they are floating away.

Developmental Adaptations:

Assist younger children in any writing or cutting, as necessary.

Alternative Activity Debrief:

Discuss how, once the thoughts were cut up and rearranged, their meanings disappear, and instead, they can become beautiful art. Discuss how we can "play" with the words we tell ourselves in order to help thoughts not feel so hurtful and sticky inside of our minds.

80TH BIRTHDAY PARTY EXERCISE (10 MINUTES)

Materials:

- None

Description:

The 80th birthday party is a technique that can help the youth explore what they value (Harris, 2009). Have the youth imagine they are celebrating their eightieth birthday. They get to select three people who will stand up and give a speech about them, and what the youth stood for in their life. This is the youth's fantasy, so they can include people who likely may not still be alive at the time of this party (e.g., the youth's parents or grandparents) or who may not exist yet in the youth's life (e.g., a future life partner, spouse, colleague, or child). The descriptors that are included in the "speeches" are often the areas the youth most values.

PRACTITIONER: *Today, we are going to have you all imagine your eightieth birthday parties. Take a moment to imagine the scene, with the decorations, the food, and the music. Now imagine that three different people stand up to make speeches about you. This is your fantasy birthday party, so these people can be anyone you want, including people who have already died, such as a grandparent or parent you don't think will still be alive when you turn eighty, or a future child, boss, or best friend. This is your fantasy, so include anyone whom you truly care about, OK?*

Now imagine the first person you have chosen gets up and makes a short speech about you, just a few sentences. The speech will be about what you stand for in life and what you mean to them. Go ahead and take a few moments to think about that and tell me what they will say.

Allow some time for the youth to think about this and let them share what would be said in these speeches. Write down some key words mentioned by each youth by their name on a notepad so that these comments can be further reflected on later in the session.

PRACTITIONER: *The things that you shared from these speeches are likely to be things that you value in your life or things you want to accomplish. Let's talk about that, and how knowing these values and goals can be helpful to you in this moment.*

Developmental Adaptations:

This activity is likely too advanced for younger children. Instead, the Children's Values Worksheet (Play Attune, 2021) could be utilized in order to better assist young children in their values identification. This worksheet can be found at: https://langlade.extension. wisc.edu/files/2020/07/Childrens-Values-Worksheet.pdf

Activity Debrief:

The practitioner can discuss with the youth what specific actions and behaviors can be taken to support the values listed in the "speeches." Goals can then be formulated in the areas that are most valued and actions to reach these goals can then be considered.

ACTIVITY: VALUES REFINEMENT (10 MINUTES)

Materials:

• Values List Handout 5.2

Description:

Following completion of the 80th birthday party exercise, you can support the youth in completing the Values List handout to further expand upon and refine their core values (Harris, 2009). Some of the most commonly held values for youth fall in the following areas: family relationships; peer relationships; academics; hobbies and activities; sports; spirituality; citizenship; and health and physical well-being (adapted from Hayes & Smith, 2005). Other areas can be added, as appropriate, particularly those that may have been identified in the 80th birthday party exercise.

Have the youth identify those value areas that are most important to them by rank ordering them on the Values List (Handout 5.2). Discuss specific actions that align with each of the three top rated value areas. Following are examples of actions:

- Family relationships: getting along with parents, siblings, and other family members; helping around the house.
- Peer relationships: being supportive; being kind; being a good listener; sharing.
- Academics: being helpful to other students; being a good listener; completing work; being focused; being respectful.
- Hobbies and activities: being creative; trying new activities; completing projects; contributing to the group; being a leader.
- Sports: being a good teammate; cooperating with others; giving it your best; challenging yourself.
- Spirituality: attending services; practicing spirituality in various ways according to beliefs.
- Health and fitness: eating healthy; exercising; getting enough sleep.

Developmental Adaptations:

Younger group members are encouraged to draw pictures of the things that are most important to them. Prompt group members to reference their completed Children's Value Worksheet and identify things that are important to them that weren't on that worksheet and/or draw pictures that further illustrate values they identified on the worksheet. You can give them suggestions of what to draw, such as "My Family," "My Friends," "My School," and so on. After members have drawn these areas, go around the circle and have each member describe what they drew. Suggest ideas of how these things we value can be supported with the things we do (e.g., if family is drawn, discuss ways the youth can get along with family members and be a helpful member of the family). These identified values can then be used in the next activity, Road Map to Success.

Activity Debrief:

Discuss how short-term and long-term goals can be created based on the values ranked as most important and the corresponding specific actions identified. Note that these values/actions will be used in the next activity, Road Map to Success.

ACTIVITY: ROAD MAP TO SUCCESS (10 MINUTES)

Materials:

- Road Map to Success Diagram (Handout 5.3)

Description:

The Road Map to Success can aid members in setting short-term and long-term goals. On the map, the youth will write next to the "road signs" actions that will help them meet their values-based goals, as found through the 80th Birthday Party and the Values List activities.

Hand out the Road Map to Success Diagram (Handout 5.3). Tell the members to choose one value that they rated highly on their values list to use on their roadmaps. Once a value has been chosen, discuss the specific actions that are necessary to support that value. Then create short-term and long-term goals based on these actions.

Give an example. If the value is "academics," the specific action identified may have been "to improve as a student." A short-term goal might be, "organize my backpack"; a medium-term goal might be, "use my planner to check off assignments and remember upcoming tests over the next 2 weeks." A long-term goal might be, "finish papers before deadlines and study for tests over the weekends." These could all be added to road signs 1 to 5, respectively.

Developmental Adaptations:

Simplify directions for younger children, though goals can still be set based on the developmental adaptations found in the Values List activity.

Activity Debrief:

Encourage youth to share examples of their values, specific actions, and short-term/long-term goals with the larger group. Discuss any challenges group members encountered in identifying short-term and long-term goals. Provide support in refining these goals, as necessary.

Closing Activity: Home Practice

Encourage youth to take one step toward their short-term goals before the next session. Encourage youth to continue using their 4x8 breaths and other mindfulness and cognitive defusion skills discussed to date.

Session 7: When Roadblocks Happen

Objectives:

- To aid the youth in predicting challenges that will arise in their lives
- To prevent relapse
- To review mindfulness and acceptance practices

Session Materials Needed:

- Mountain Handout (5.4)
- Sticky notes with pre-written sayings, such as "You will never make it!," "Just give up!," and "Why even try?!"
- Blank paper and a pen
- Optional Activity: finger paints and butcher paper

Opening Statement:

PRACTITIONER: *Today, we are going to talk about how, when we make progress toward our goals, roadblocks can come up that make us feel like we haven't gotten anywhere. It can be really discouraging when that happens. We will talk about how to keep moving toward our goals, even when unexpected roadblocks appear.*

HOME PRACTICE REVIEW (5 MINUTES)

Open the discussion around members' short-term goals identified last week and what, if any, progress they made in achieving these goals. If some members did not take a step toward their goals, discuss how they can proceed on their roadmap's first short-term goal over the next week.

OPENING ACTIVITY: CLIMBING THE MOUNTAIN (5 MINUTES)

Materials:

- Mountain Handout (Handout 5.4)

Description:

A useful metaphor for setbacks is climbing a mountain. Give the Mountain Handout (5.4) to each child.

PRACTITIONER: *Often mountain climbers experience setbacks along their way. The adjustments they make, such as taking a step back, taking in a deep breath, and getting different footing, can assist them in feeling more stable and help them to move even higher toward their intended goal. Has anyone ever had that experience on a hike or when you were climbing something?*

Wait for responses. Discuss how often things don't always go according to plan, and sometimes we need to adjust our path.

Developmental Adaptations:

Modify the script to use more simplified language, if needed.

Activity Debrief:

This mountain analogy can be used to help group members more reasonably assess setbacks. They do not have to be called failures. Instead, a change on their path may help them make even more progress in the end. Challenges can be understood by the youth as "opportunities." Using their mindfulness and acceptance skills can help them take advantage of challenges.

ACTIVITY: SWAMP (5 MINUTES)

Materials:

* Only if conducting the optional activity (see materials list for Swamp Art Activity).

Description:

As discussed in the last activity, unexpected circumstances can be encountered on hikes. We have to decide how to react to these challenges: turn back and give up, stay stuck, or move through it. The following script uses the swamp (Harris, 2009) as a metaphor for challenges encountered toward goal completion.

PRACTITIONER: *As we move toward our goals, problems can crop up. We usually don't have control over these problems, but we can control how we react to them. Let's imagine that your goal is to make it to the top of a mountain you have always wanted to climb. Take a few moments right now to take a few deep breaths, then imagine this mountain.*
Lead youth in four, 4x8 breaths.
PRACTITIONER: *So, imagine you are walking along your path toward the mountain, and you are feeling pretty good about your progress. The sun is out, and the air feels good. Now imagine right as you get up to the base of the mountain, right before you are going to make that final climb up, you stumble upon a swamp. This swamp encircles the entire mountain, so there is no*

way to avoid it. *It's gooey and green and you hadn't expected it to be there at all. It is a big surprise! So now you have to decide – What do you do? Do you throw your hands up and give up on your goal?*

Wait for members to respond. Suggest that they really wanted to get to the top of the mountain so much that they decided to stick with it.

PRACTITIONER: *OK, would you wade into the swamp and hang out in it? Swim around and decide to stay in it? Perhaps do the backstroke?*

Wait for reaction here (often laughter).

PRACTITIONER: *Of course not! There is one other choice you can make. You can tell yourself, "Well, here is a swamp. This is not going how I thought it would, and I had not expected this swamp. But I will accept that it is here, and move through it as easily as I can, without it getting so sticky that I can't get out of it, and also not give up on my goal."*

Developmental Adaptations:

This technique can be used with almost all ages, incorporating the use of visuals or an art project for younger children (e.g., the use of finger paints to create the goal on the hill and the swamp surrounding it, as depicted in the optional activity of Swamp Art described later).

Activity Debrief:

Discuss how often we encounter "swamps" when going toward our goals. It is not what we expected, nor what we wanted. But we can just accept the reality that they are there and move through them.

OPTIONAL ACTIVITY: SWAMP ART (15 MINUTES)

Materials:

- Large butcher paper or poster paper with a mountain drawn on it
- Paints appropriate for finger painting
- Wet wipes for clean-up

Directions:

In this activity, group members will create their own swamp with finger paints. This swamp will be a metaphor for how everyone encounters challenges along their paths.

Ask members what goal they would like to work on. The group leader should now know the children from prior sessions and can give them suggestions for goals (e.g., to make more friends, or to feel calmer). These goals can be written at the top of the mountain on the butcher paper.

Instruct members to together paint a "swamp" around the base of the mountain. Mixing the colors together is encouraged, as this often makes the swamp a brownish-green in the end. Give members about 5 minutes to paint the swamp together. Before beginning the debrief, hand out wet wipes for the children to clean off their fingers.

Developmental Adaptations:

None. This activity is appropriate for any age group, though particularly geared toward younger children.

Activity Debrief:

Discuss how often we encounter "swamps" when moving toward our goals. If our goal was to climb to the top of the mountain, we may feel discouraged if we come to a swamp. It is not what we expected, nor what we wanted, but we can just accept that it is there and move through it. This lets us be on our way instead of getting stuck in it, swimming around in it, or giving up on our goal. Prompt the group members to describe how they can "move through the swamp" relevant to their specific goals.

ACTIVITY: PASSENGERS ON THE BUS (15 MINUTES)

Materials:

- 3–4 chairs
- Sticky notes with pre-written sayings, such as "You will never make it!," "Just give up!," and "Why even try?!"
- Blank paper and a pen

Description:

In the passengers on the bus metaphor, the youth is the bus driver, and the passengers are their thoughts. Even though the passengers may be noisily shouting to go various ways, the driver can continue to move toward their goal (Hayes et al., 2012).

Set up the chairs so there is one chair in the front (the driver), and two to three chairs behind it, as if in a bus. In this activity, the members will role play being passengers on a bus. The passengers will try to distract the driver by saying negative thoughts. The goal of this role play is to show group members that the driver controls the bus, not the passengers, and how easy it is to get distracted by negative thoughts when trying to pursue a goal.

It is best if the group leader begins as the bus driver. The bus driver will write down on a blank sheet of paper the goal they want to move toward. An example could be for the group leader to write for themselves, "To be more organized," "To be more social," or "To learn how to ____ (fill in the blank, such as "speak Spanish," or "play the piano"). Tape this goal to a wall in front of the bus driver (as if the bus would be driving toward the goal). Ask for volunteers or select group members to come and be the passengers for the first round.

The group leader will randomly hand out sayings on sticky notes to the passengers. The leader explains that the passengers' job is to distract the bus driver by calling out these thoughts. The bus driver then takes their seat and pretends to begin driving. Here is when the passengers begin to yell out the unhelpful thoughts on the notes. At first the bus driver should role play the driver giving attention to the passengers; perhaps the passengers make the driver turn around, make the driver stop the bus and get out of their seat. Maybe the driver stops to try to throw a passenger off the bus. Have the driver talk to themselves out loud, such as "I can't focus on driving with these passengers," "Maybe I should just give up," and "I need these passengers off my bus!"

Turn to the remaining group members who are not currently passengers and ask for advice. Work in the ideas of using the mindfulness and acceptance techniques learned throughout the group, such as taking in some deep 4x8 breaths and using acceptance language, such as, "I hear you back there, but instead of being distracted by you, I am going to accept you are there and just keep driving toward my goal."

Once the leader has modeled for the group the idea behind the role play, group members can take turns as the bus driver and write their goals on a piece of paper. Other group members can play the passengers. Give suggestions and advice to the bus driver as a consultant, help the driver use mindfulness and acceptance tools to keep moving toward their goal.

Developmental Adaptations:

If a role play seems too disruptive or challenging for younger students, spend more time on the optional activity of the Swamp Art. Another alternative activity for young children would be to watch a short online video on the metaphor. Here are several examples, though others could be used as well.

- www.youtube.com/watch?v=ztlo50h0T2Q
- www.youtube.com/watch?v=Z29ptSuoWRc

Activity Debrief:

Discuss with the members how it felt to be the bus driver. Acknowledge how often our difficult thoughts can be distracting and make it harder to reach our goals. Review mindfulness and acceptance tools to aid members in changing their relationship and attachment to these thoughts.

CLOSING ACTIVITY: HOME PRACTICE

Encourage members over the next week to practice using their mindfulness and acceptance tools when they hear their own "passengers" in their minds.

Session 8: Wrapping Up

Objectives:

• To review key components of mindfulness and acceptance practices
• To celebrate successes
• To create a plan for further services, if needed

Session Materials Needed:

• Food or drink, as appropriate. Take any food allergies into account for members.
• Mindfulness and Acceptance Strategy Cards (Handout 5.5 cut into individual cards)

Opening Statement:

PRACTITIONER: *Today is our last session together in this group. We are going to review some things we have worked on, as well as celebrate our time together and your accomplishments.*

OPENING ACTIVITY: RETURN TO OUR 5 SENSES (10 MINUTES)

Now that the members have had eight sessions of mindfulness and acceptance work, the technique below incorporates the 5 Senses technique with other acceptance tools.

PRACTITIONER: *We are going to use our five senses to help us to be right here in this moment. We will be using our hearing, seeing, tasting, touching, and smelling to just be here in this room.*

As we have learned, thinking is not a sense, but sometimes we think about things so much that we miss what is actually happening around us. Often the way to really know what is actually happening is by using our five senses.

We will start by taking in a few deep 4x8 breaths, as we have been working on. A deep breath in through our nose to the count of four, hold it briefly, then out to the count of eight. Good, let's do another.

Model with the youth taking in these deep breaths. Take four deep breaths with them.

Good, now, either soften your eyes, without focusing hard on any one thing, and look toward the floor or, if you are comfortable with it, close your eyes.

Model this for the members.

As we continue to take in those deep 4 by 8 breaths, we will turn our attention to what we are hearing right now in the room.

Note for the members what sounds can be heard either inside or outside. The following sample can be modified as to what is being heard in that moment.

Perhaps you hear the sound of the air conditioner, or the clock ticking. You may hear sounds outside the room, like people talking or traffic going by. Just focus on your deep breaths, and what you are hearing right now.

When a thought comes into the room, put that thought in a bubble and let that go; open your mental hands and let the thought float away. Then focus again on your deep 4x8 breaths and what you are hearing right now in this room.

Good, now notice the weight of your body in your chair. Notice the solidness of the floor underneath your feet. Note the temperature of the air on your face and hands. Just be right here. Notice the parts of your back that are touching the chair and the parts of your back that are not, and the difference between those. We will continue to take our deep breaths in to the count of four, and out to the count of eight.

Notice if you have any taste on your tongue. Note if you can smell any smells or scents in the room.

Now open your eyes and look around the room. You may notice that colors seem brighter, and lines on objects are sharper and clearer. Perhaps you notice something in the room that you had not noticed before.

Good, and we will take in one last deep breath, and let it out.

Developmental Adaptations:

The cadence of the breaths can be altered so that they are not so elongated for young children.

Activity Debrief:

Ask the members how that exercise was for them, and have them describe what it was like to use their five senses in this way. Ask them if they noticed something in the room (i.e., what they heard or saw) that they had not noticed when they came into the group that day. Ask members if it is easier now to not feel so distracted by thoughts. Encourage members to reflect on how this exercise felt different completing it today compared to the first time they did it earlier in the group. Emphasize how any improvements are a result of practice and encourage continued practice to further master this technique. Discuss other ways to help "open their mental hands" to let thoughts go.

HOME PRACTICE REVIEW (5 MINUTES)

Discuss with members whether they used their mindfulness and acceptance tools when they heard their own "passengers" in their minds or noticed "swamps" over the last week.

RETURN TO MINDFUL EATING ACTIVITY (10 MINUTES)

Materials:

• Food and drink item brought to session

Description:

In this activity, youth will again explore mindful eating. The following script can be adapted for whatever food and drink items are brought to the session to celebrate the day.

PRACTITIONER: *Today, we are going to use mindful eating to enjoy the first bite of the food I brought in to share today. While holding the food in your hand, we are again going to pretend like we are visitors from another planet and are experiencing this food for the first time. We are going to use all of our five senses to investigate this object.*

Model holding the food between your index finger and thumb, bringing it up to your face.

Look at the object as you hold it in your fingers. Notice what it looks like. Is it shiny or dull, bumpy or smooth? What color is it? Does the light catch the object on some areas differently than others? What does the weight of it feel like in your hand?

Now we are going to use our sense of smell to smell the object. Breathe deeply as you hold your object under your nose. Notice if you can smell any scents as you breath in deeply. Good, let's try that again.

Model breathing in deeply as you hold the food item under your nose.

Now, place the object on your tongue and just hold it there. What does it feel like? Can you taste anything? Now slowly chew your object, starting with just one bite. Can you hear any sounds as you take this bite? Does the object change form as you bite it? Is there more flavor now that you can taste?

Pause a moment while the youth chews the object.

Good, now, as you swallow the object, do you notice any taste left on your tongue?

Developmental Adaptations:

Typically, this exercise does not need adaptation and can be used for any age range.

Activity Debrief:

Engage the youth in a discussion about the exercise. Ask how this is different from how they usually eat something. As the group continues to eat their snacks, discuss whether eating in a mindful way can leave us with a more satisfied feeling. Have the group members enjoyed the food more than if they had quickly eaten it without having awareness?

MINDFULNESS AND ACCEPTANCE CHARADES (15 MINUTES)

Materials:

* Twelve Mindfulness and Acceptance Tool Kit Cards (Handout 5.5), photocopied and cut out. Prepare one set of cards for each group member.

Description:

This activity provides a review of the tools and techniques covered over the eight-session group program. There are two ways the set of cards can be used in games. The first game is to have group members, in turn, act out a technique from a card while the other members guess the technique, as in a game of charades. The second game is to have members take turns drawing a picture of the technique, while others guess what it is, as in a game of Pictionary. Both adaptations are offered next. Note that only one deck of tool cards is used for these activities, but afterwards each member will receive their own deck. Before playing either game, the group leader can present all of the cards to the members, asking them to recall each technique. This can be an excellent review before the game.

Charades: Each member will have a turn to choose a card, get up in front of the group and act out the technique on the card. The other members guess what card they pulled. The youth acting out the technique cannot use any words when members are guessing the card. Once the card has been correctly guessed, another group member will choose a card and continue the game.

Drawing Game: Each member will have a turn to choose a card and draw the activity listed on the card. The other members guess what activity they are drawing. The student drawing cannot speak or write words when members are guessing the card. Once the card has been correctly guessed, another group member will then choose a card to draw and continue the game.

Developmental Adaptations:

Younger children may find that acting out the tools is easier than drawing them. Older youth may prefer the drawing activity. For either activity, group leaders may need to read the card quietly to the youth whose turn it is in order to ensure understanding.

Activity Debrief:

Discuss with the group how many tools and techniques they now have in their mindfulness and acceptance "tool kits." Encourage group members to share a technique that they have found to be particularly helpful to them. Review any techniques where members have questions. Hand out a set of the tool kit cards to each group member.

CLOSING ACTIVITY

Even though it is the final session, explain that the work they started with one another will go on through their use of the techniques. If anyone feels they need additional support or help, tell them to please see you after the session to discuss further services. Thank everyone for being a part of the group.

Form 5.1

Teacher Letter

FOR RECRUITING STUDENTS

Dear _____,   *Date:* _____

We are seeking students who would benefit from extra social and emotional support through participation in a small mindfulness group. The group will teach students healthy ways of coping with difficult feelings and thoughts. We are looking for your recommendations of students you think will benefit.

The group will meet every _____ for 45–50 minutes for eight sessions, starting on _____. Students will be held accountable for any schoolwork missed during the group sessions.

Please fill out and return the attached referral form no later than _____ to _____.
Feel free to copy the referral form if you have more than one student who you believe will benefit.

Thank you for your time!

Sincerely,

_____

Form 5.2

Teacher Referral Form:

MINDFULNESS AND ACT GROUP

Student's Name: _____

Teacher: _____

Grade: _____   Room: _____

1. Why do you think this student would benefit from participating in this group?

2. What skills or special talents do you see this student as having?

3. What social or emotional skills would you like to see this student develop?

Form 5.3

Parent/Guardian Permission Letter

Date:_____ Student's Name:_____

Dear Parent or Guardian,

As part of the mission to support students in their social and emotional health, we offer a variety of small groups throughout the school year. We would like to invite your child, _____, to participate in a small group experience that teaches students healthy ways of coping with difficult feelings and thoughts. These skills can be helpful for managing emotions, increasing focus in the classroom, and helping social relationships. It is our belief that all students have something to contribute and something to gain during this group experience. The group will meet for eight sessions once a week for 45–50 minutes during the school day beginning _____.

The specific meeting time will be determined with teachers to ensure the least impact on the student's academics, though students will be responsible for any work missed during the meetings. Teachers are supportive of this group experience. If you have any questions specifically about your child's academics, it is best to contact your child's teacher.

Participation in the group is voluntary and anything your child shares in the group will be kept confidential. This means that, without your written permission, we will not share anything your child shares with anyone else outside of the group. This is to help foster trust and encourage participation of the group members. However, there are certain situations wherein confidentiality must be breached, including situations where a student's safety is at risk. If you have any questions, please feel free to contact the facilitators at _____.

Sincerely,

_____
Group Facilitator

Sign, Cut and Return the Below to Your Child's Teacher

_____ **I give permission for my child, _____, to participate in the group.**

_____ **I do not give permission for my child to participate in the group.**

_____
Parent Signature

_____
Youth Signature

Form 5.4

Ready-Set-Go! Checklist

SMALL GROUP WORK

Table 5.1

Task	Date Sent/Accomplished
Create Buy-In (teachers meeting, speak with principal, etc.)	
Send out Teacher Recruitment Letter and Referral Form	
Organize List of Prospective Group Members	
Send Parent/Guardian Permission Letter	
Interview/Screen Prospective Group Members	
Determine Time/Day/Physical Setting for Group	
Review all Curriculum Sessions, Making Modifications as Necessary; Prepare Needed Materials	
Start Your Group!	

Handout 5.1 Brain Structure

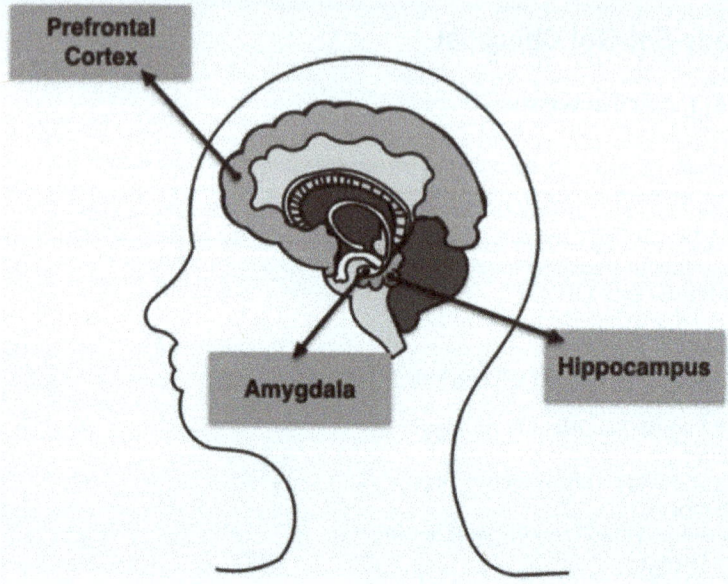

Handout 5.2

Values List Handout

Rank order the below, 1–7, in order of most importance in your life. Give an example of one way you can support this value through something you can do.

<u>**Rank**</u> <u>**Value**</u>   <u>**Example of an Action You Can Take**</u>

____   Family relationships

____   Peer relationships

____   Academics

____   Hobbies and activities

____   Spirituality

____   Citizenship

____   Health/physical well-being

Handout 5.3

Road Map to Success Diagram

Value: _____

Goals:

1: _____

2: _____

3: _____

4: _____

5: _____

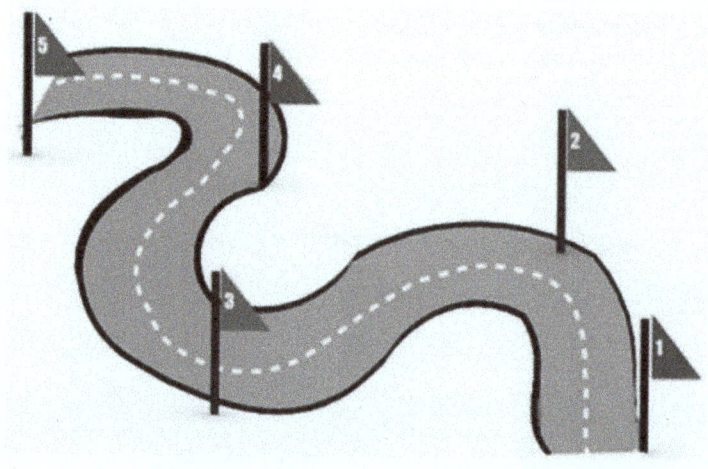

Handout 5.4

Mountain Handout

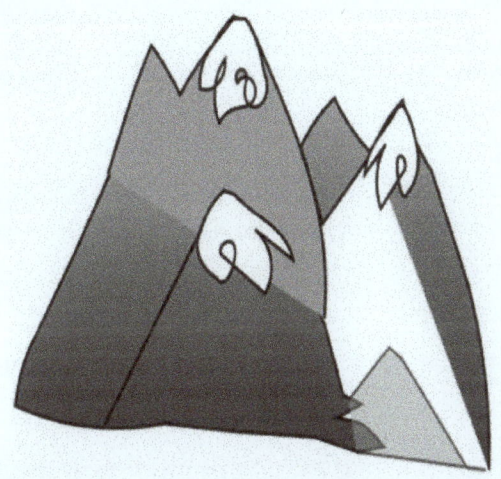

Handout 5.5

Mindfulness and Acceptance Tool Kit Cards

5 Senses Activity	Chinese Finger Traps	Passengers on the Bus
Thought Globe Activity	4 x 8 Breaths	Climbing the Mountain Metaphor
Clipboard Activity	Thought Bubbles	80th Birthday Party
Swamp Metaphor	Mindful Eating	Sunglasses Metaphor

Cut along each line to make 12 cards total.

References

Center for Substance Abuse Treatment. (1999). *Treatment improvement protocol (TIP) series, No. 34. Brief interventions and brief therapies for substance abuse.* Substance Abuse and Mental Health Services Administration.

Cooley, L. (Ed.). (2009). *The power of groups: Solution-focused group counseling in schools.* Corwin.

DiOrio, R. (2010). *What does it mean to be present?* Little Pickle Stories.

Gerrity, D. A., & DeLucia-Waack, J. L. (2006). Effectiveness of groups in the schools. *The Journal for Specialists in Group Work, 32*(1), 97–106.

Haen, C., & Aronson, S. (2016). *Handbook of child and adolescent group therapy: A practitioner's reference.* Taylor & Francis.

Harris, R. (2009). *ACT made simple: A quick start guide to ACT basics and beyond.* New Harbinger Publication.

Hayes, S. C., & Smith, S. (2005). *Get out of your mind and into your life: The new acceptance and commitment therapy.* New Harbinger Publications.

Hayes, S. C., Strosahl, K. D., & Wilson, K. G. (2012). *Acceptance and commitment therapy: An experiential approach to behavior change* (2nd ed.). Guilford Press.

Hoag, M. J., & Burlingame, G. M. (2009). Evaluating the effectiveness of child and adolescent group treatment: A meta-analytic review. *Journal of Clinical Child Psychology, 26*(3), 234–246.

Kulic, K. R., Horne, A. M., & Dagley, J. C. (2004). A comprehensive review of prevention groups for children and adolescents. *Group Dynamics, Theory, Research and Practice, 8*(2), 139–151.

Nance, A. J. (2016). *Puppy mind.* Plum Blossom.

Piaget, J. (1969). *The psychology of the child.* Basic Books.

Play Attune. (2021). *Children's value worksheet.* https://langlade.extension.wisc.edu/files/2020/07/Childrens-Values-Worksheet.pdf

Tichener, E. B. (1916). *A text-book of psychology.* Macmillan.

Yalom, I. D., & Leszcz, M. (2005). *The theory and practice of group psychotherapy* (5th ed.). Basic Books.

6 Mindfulness and ACT Strategies for Classroom and School-Wide Programming

Roadmap to Chapter 6:
   This chapter considers aspects of running large, classroom and school-wide groups with youth. Specifically, it covers:

- mindfulness techniques that can be integrated into the broader school day
- classroom-wide mindfulness and acceptance practices
- specific mindfulness programs for the classroom or school-wide.

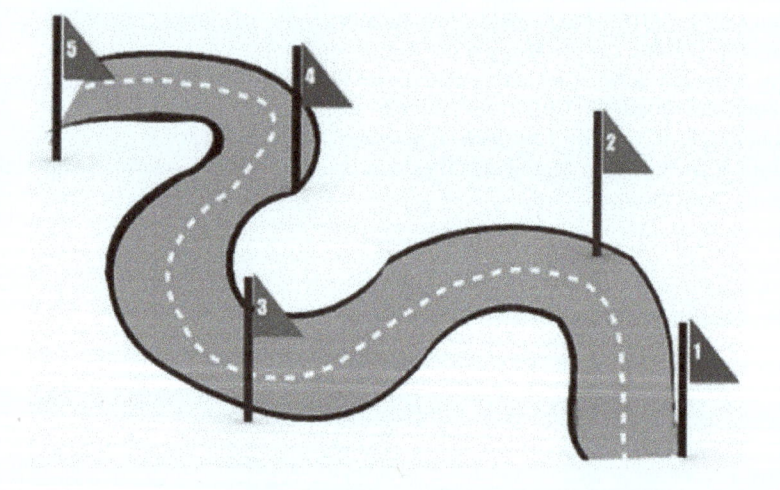

As reviewed in Chapter 2, mindfulness practices can reduce stress, improve emotion regulation, and contribute to overall mental health (Hanson & Mendius, 2009; National Center for Complementary and Integrative Medicine, 2017). These practices have also been shown to boost academic functioning and performance in the classroom (Roodenrys et al., 2017). The addition of acceptance practices can further

DOI: 10.4324/9781003318101-6

reduce student stress levels (Livheim et al., 2014). Given the positive benefits of mindfulness and acceptance practices for students and teachers, consider adapting these methods for wider audiences. This chapter overviews classroom and school-wide mindfulness and acceptance practices. We begin with suggestions for incorporating individual techniques into the classroom and then review specific classroom and school-wide programs.

Integrating Mindfulness Practices into the Classroom

Many of the mindfulness techniques covered in Chapter 3 can be woven in various ways throughout the regular school day. These activities can be adapted for use with any age or grade level, by simply altering the language used by the teacher or practitioner. Table 6.1 summarizes the strategies reviewed later.

Mindful Breathing

As overviewed in Chapters 2 and 3, mindful breathing can lead to emotional well-being and increased cognitive performance. One simple practice is to have students begin their school day by taking in four deep, 4x8 breaths when the final bell rings. This can lead to youth feeling more centered and grounded as they begin their academic day. Teachers can also have students take in 4x8 breaths as they sit down to complete an exam or give a presentation. Often students feel anxious before such tasks. Mindful breaths can calm their sympathetic nervous systems (SNS)

Table 6.1 Summary of ideas for classroom mindfulness-based strategies in this chapter.

Strategies	Definitions
Mindful Breathing	Prompt students to take 4x8 breaths throughout the day (e.g., start of school day, before tests, if class becomes restless, etc.).
Mindful Language	Continue to use mindful language throughout the school day with students.
Mindful Eating	Encourage students to use all five senses when eating food.
Heartfulness	Encourage students to engage in heartfulness during their school days to aid in empathy and perspective taking.
Mindful Transitions	Use mindfulness activities during times of transition throughout the school day.
Mindful Corner	Provide a quiet space for youth designated for mindfulness in the classroom.

and allow them to have greater access to logical reason and memory. It can be an effective tool for boosting well-being and performance.

Mindful Language

The Take 5 tool in Chapter 3 (Form 3.8) can be adapted, with the teacher prompting the whole class to notice each of their five senses. This exercise can be particularly helpful in grounding the class if it seems unsettled or distracted. Once introduced to mindfulness and some of the techniques, the teacher can simply use terms like "mindful feet" or "mindful body" if a child needs to be reminded of personal space or activity. If a teacher or staff member notes a child using negative labeling or "I am" statements, as overviewed in Chapter 4, these statements can be reframed for the child as, "You are having the thought that . . . ." Remind the child that those are just thoughts, then help the child to refocus on the present moment or the task at hand.

Mindful Snacking

You can lead youth at snack time in the mindful eating activity, as described in Chapter 3. Use the five senses to increase presence for their first bite of food. Even young children can benefit from mindfully eating the first bite of their snack or lunch. Mindful eating practices can be encouraged classroom-wide, or even lunchroom-wide!

Heartfulness

Heartfulness means having a warm, connected relationship with whatever is happening in our experience, external or internal. Encouraging students to engage in heartfulness aids in developing empathy, kindness, and perspective taking (Sofer, 2016). It can be used with any grade level. As noted in Chapter 3, gratitude journaling can focus youth on positive values and experiences, such as noting three things they are grateful for. This can also help students with setting intentions and goals for their day, such as taking specific actions toward goals in their gratitude areas. Encouraging mindful listening to others can also be a heartful practice and can aid positive social skills and interactions. This can be easily accomplished during "circle time" or other times during the school day when students face one another and share. Another technique for heartfulness is for the teacher to note at the start of the school day those students who are absent and lead the students present in the following simple meditation: say the absent student's name, then say, "May you be happy, may you be healthy, may you be well." This encourages youth to care for their community and have empathy toward those who may be ill.

Mindful Transitions

Transitions can be very challenging times of the school day, especially when moving from a less structured activity, such as lunch or recess, into a more structured activity, such as math or reading. The use of mindful breathing or mindful listening can be helpful to focus students on the present moment. In another brief activity, have youth take their seats upon entering a room and then quietly listen to a bell that is rung. Instruct them to silently raise their hands when they can no longer perceive the sound. This can be an excellent transition activity and leaves them present and focused for the next task.

Mindful Corner

Setting up a "mindful corner" of the classroom or playground can be useful for some students who need a more structured environmental context for bringing themselves into the present moment. Depending on the setting, provide a quiet space youth can use to control for over-stimulation and aid in mindful presence. Have a few visual reminders around the physical space, such as pictures or words reminding youth of the 4x8 breathing technique and the 5 Senses technique.

Cognitive Defusion

One example of a metaphor that can be used classroom-wide is a spider web representing our minds. The class can be told that getting stuck in the web is similar to getting stuck in their thoughts. Just as one part of the web may "catch us," so can our thoughts and this can prevent us from moving forward in our value-driven goals. This can be further expanded to represent cognitive defusion since the spider can walk around the web without getting entangled. The class can then discuss how they can become more like the spider and less like a fly. These metaphors, combined with the creative activity of making a spider web (e.g., drawing it or making it using stretched cotton balls, etc.) can be an effective way of teaching cognitive defusion, even to younger children (Szabo & Dixon, 2016).

A Sampling of Specific Mindfulness Programs

Many schools consider using structured, published programs when starting a classroom or school-wide practice. Table 6.2 lists a sampling of specific mindfulness programs that can be accessed for school use. For each program, the table gives its targeted age and developmental range, along with a brief description of implementation and research support. The text then gives a more in-depth look at each program. Note that the

Table 6.2 Evidence-based mindfulness programs.

Name	Target ages	Number and/ or frequency of sessions	Focus of sessions	Evidence of efficacy
Mindful Schools (2019)	5–18	2–3, 15-minute sessions per week for 10–15 weeks	Through professional or trained educator-led sessions, Mindful Schools focuses on building attention, self-regulation, and empathy by teaching youth mindful: breathing, sensory experience, and emotions and thoughts.	Evidence suggests that the Mindful Schools curriculum is effective in improving attention and class participation in students and mindfulness in teachers (Mindful Schools, 2015b).
Inner Explorer (Houlihan & Bakosh, 2011)	3–18	Daily, 5–10-minute lessons for 10–18 weeks	Using pre-recorded audio instruction in home and at school, Inner Explorer improves emotional regulation and self-awareness through mindfulness-based stress reduction techniques.	The Inner Explorer program has primarily been examined in elementary school age youth, and has been found to be effective in improving academic scores, including math and science scores (Bakosh et al., 2018), as well as improvements in reading scores (Bakosh et al., 2014). In addition, the program was found to reduce negative classroom behavioral events (Bakosh et al., 2014).
MindUP (2003)	3–14	15 lessons total, practiced several times a day	Focuses on enhancing student self-awareness, focused attention, self-regulation, and stress reduction through engaging in didactic lessons, deep breathing, and attentive listening.	The MindUP program has been examined in elementary and middle school age youth, and was found to be effective in improving student characteristics, including optimism, mindfulness, empathy, and perspective taking (Schonert-Reichl et al., 2015) In addition, Schonert-Reichl and Lawlor (2010) found that after participating in the program, teachers rated students higher in social exchanges and optimism and reported fewer disruptive behaviors.

Program	Age	Frequency	Description	Research
Still Quiet Place (Saltzman, 2014)	5–18	Once weekly, 8 weeks long	Goal is to improve behavioral and emotional self-regulation, and general well-being by teaching youth mindfulness, breathwork, body-scanning, and loving kindness practices. Additional home practice is encouraged through guided audio meditations.	Saltzman and Goldin (2008) found that in a self-referred nonclinical community sample of 24 families (31 children, and 27 parents) those who engaged in the Still Quiet Place curriculum showed improvements in attention, mood, and metacognitive domains (compassion and mindfulness), compared to wait-list controls.
Stressed Teens (2019)	13–18	8 weeks total	Reduces stress in teens by using mindfulness-based stress reduction activities, including meditation, body scans, mindful awareness, and heartfulness activities.	Biegel et al. (2009) found that in a sample of 102, 14–18-year-olds former or current outpatient psychiatric care patients, those in the Stressed Teens program showed reductions in anxiety, depressive and somatic symptoms, and improved self-esteem and sleep quality, compared to controls. In addition, 45% showed positive diagnostic change, whereas almost none of the control participants did.
Mindful Life Project (2021)	5–13	Once per week, 25-minute lessons	Teaches students self-awareness, impulse control, self-regulation, resiliency, and confidence through mindfulness, yoga, expressive arts, and hip-hop/dance.	Unpublished internal research suggests that after participating in the program 83% of teachers noticed improvement in their students' self-awareness, and 71% in attentional abilities (Mindful Life Project, 2019). Additionally, suspension rates were lower in participating schools (Mindful Life Project, 2019). Crockett-Chaney (2018), in an unpublished dissertation, found that 42 fourth graders participating in the program showed increased mindfulness skills, improved self-regulation, and more positive classroom behavior, compared to wait-list controls.
Wellness Works in Schools (2017)	3–18	8–15 lessons	Focuses on enhancing mental, emotional, physical, and social health in youth through mindfulness training.	Unpublished internal research suggests that following participation in the program, 94% of teachers noticed an improvement in student attention, 82% of students reported that they could better regulate their behavior, and 76% showed increased ability to manage stress and regulate emotions (Wellness Works in Schools, 2017).

(Continued)

Name	Target ages	Number and/or frequency of sessions	Focus of sessions	Evidence of efficacy
Center for Resilience (2018)	5–18	30-minute sessions, twice weekly for 32 weeks	This program is aligned with the five CASEL (2019) competencies of self-awareness, self-management, relationship skills, social awareness, and responsible decision-making. Students are taught breathwork, yoga, mindfulness movement, and meditation.	No formal studies have been undertaken examining the efficacy of this program. However, unpublished internal evaluation suggests that the program led to "dramatic reductions in student and teacher stress; bullying; and behavior-related visits to the principal's office" (Center for Resilience, 2018).
Master Mind Academy (Innovation Research and Training, 2014)	9–11	15 minutes daily for 4 weeks	Uses teacher led lessons focusing on teaching mindfulness and substance abuse prevention through weekly mindfulness topics of awareness of the body, feelings, thoughts, and relationships. Additional homework activities, called "investigations" are encouraged.	Parker et al. (2014) examined the efficacy of the Master Mind Academy in sample of 111 elementary school students across two school sites. Participants compared to controls showed improvements in executive functioning, and reductions in aggression and social problems. In addition, females showed reductions in anxiety symptoms and males showed marginal increases in self-control abilities. No significant differences were found between groups for intentions to use substances.
Inner Kids Program (Greenland, 2016)	5–18	N/A	Through an online continuing education course and curated free-to-use materials focusing on mindfulness acceptance practices (MAPS) educators can learn to help promote six essential life skills in students, including Quieting, Focusing, Seeing, Reframing, Caring, and Connecting.	No studies currently exist on the Inner Kids program specifically. However, Flook et al. (2010) examined the MAPS from the Inner Kids program in a sample of 64 children ages 7–9. The study found that children with low executive functioning pre-intervention showed executive functioning in the average range post-intervention.

programs overviewed in this chapter are not intended to be exhaustive, but instead a sampling of available programs.

Mindful Schools

Mindful Schools (Mindful Schools, 2015a) is a widely used program emphasizing attention building, self-regulation, and empathy development for youth grades K–12. Two age-adapted curricula were developed: K–5 (ages 5–12) and 6–12 (ages 12–17). Lessons are taught in 15-minute sessions, two to three times a week. Specific skills included in the curricula include mindful breathing, mindful sensory experiences, and mindful emotions and thoughts. Initially, Mindful Schools sent professionals into the schools to run the sessions. More recently, however, educators have been trained in their own mindfulness practices, and then teach the skills to their students. The facilitator's training can be offered as a six-week online course or an in-person weekend training. A 10-month training is also offered to those who would like to be certified as a Mindful Schools facilitator.

Though widely used, there are only a handful of research studies on the Mindful Schools curriculum. A small 2010 pilot study found that the Mindful Schools curriculum, when used with 18 minority children at a summer camp, showed significantly more reduction in depressive symptoms than in the control group (Liehr & Diaz, 2010). In a study by Black and Fernando (2014), 409 lower-income and ethnically diverse children in kindergarten through sixth grade were exposed to either five weeks or 12 weeks of the Mindful Schools curriculum. Results from pre- to post-assessment showed that teachers reported improved classroom behavior of their students (i.e., paying attention, self-control, participation in activities, and caring and respect for others). This lasted up to seven weeks post-intervention for both groups, with overall improvements not bolstered by the addition of extra sessions, except for paying attention. These findings are limited due to the lack of a true control group and the impact of teacher expectancy effects, as it was the teachers who both implemented the program and assessed the outcome. However, these findings do suggest that mindfulness training might, at the very least, benefit teacher-based perceptions of improved classroom behavior. This has practice implications for improving the classroom learning environment for lower-income and ethnically diverse children. In a large, randomized control study, the University of California, Davis used the Mindful Schools curriculum with 937 children and 47 teachers in three Oakland public elementary schools. Findings showed statistically significant improvements in student attention and participation in class activities compared to the control group at the three-month follow up. Additionally, teachers who were the facilitators of the curriculum reported significantly increased mindfulness compared to the control teachers (Mindful Schools, 2015b). However, effect sizes across measures were relatively small and expectancy effects could again have complicated the results. Further research is warranted on this program.

Website for Mindful Schools: *www.mindfulschools.org*

Inner Explorer

The Inner Explorer (Houlihan & Bakosh, 2011) program is based on mindfulness-based stress reduction (MBSR; Kabat-Zinn, 2003) techniques, and emphasizes emotional regulation and self-awareness. The targeted age and developmental ranges are separated into four strands: preschool/kindergarten, elementary, middle school, and high school. The Inner Explorer program does not require extensive outside training or a facilitator; the materials are presented by recorded audio, with teachers and students listening to the guided daily practice together. Additionally, a parent or caretaker "Tune In" is offered via a free app (upon school purchase of the program) so families can listen to the same program as their children each day. A home edition for practice over breaks or for summer use is included to maintain continuity of skills practice throughout the year (Houlihan & Bakosh, 2011).

In a study examining the effects of the Inner Explorer program in a sample of 337 students at two elementary schools, results were mixed. At the first school, the main effect of the MBSR intervention was statistically significant for grades in Math ($p = .05$), Social Studies ($p = .008$), and on overall GPA scores ($p = .01$). For the second school, the main effect of the intervention was statistically significant for Math ($p = .001$) but none of the main effects on other grades reached statistical significance. Given the technology of Inner Explorer, teachers implemented the mindfulness-based instruction with fidelity and without the need for hiring experts outside of the school. A lack of a control group limits the findings of this study (Bakosh et al., 2018). In another study that did use a control group, eight third grade classrooms at two elementary schools used the Inner Explorer program with their students for eight weeks, including daily 10-minute audio recorded mindfulness sessions. It found significant differences in reading and science scores between the two groups when controlling for pre-intervention grades. Additionally, marked reductions in behavioral events, such as classroom disruptions and suspensions, were recorded for the treatment group, while the control group had an increase in such events. However, a lack of randomization and teacher expectation bias limit the findings of this study (Bakosh et al., 2014). Additional research using randomized control groups and more rigorous methodology is necessary.

Website for Inner Explorer: https://innerexplorer.org/

MindUP

The MindUP (2003) program is designed to be implemented in a class-room setting and provides separate sets of lessons for three grade levels: preschool through second; third through fifth; and sixth through eighth. Fifteen lessons are delivered; the core mindfulness practices of deep breathing and attentive listening are practiced several times a day. The practices in MindUP parallel the competencies included in the Collaborative for Academic, Social, and Emotional Learning (CASEL, 2019) and are designed to enhance students' self-awareness, focused attention, self-regulation, and stress reduction.

In an evaluation of the MindUP program, 246 fourth to seventh graders were assigned to either the intervention or a control group. After 10 weeks of lessons, youth in the MindUP intervention group rated themselves as significantly more optimistic, along with higher teacher rated student competencies in social exchanges, attention, and emotional awareness. Teacher rated student aggression and oppositional behavior decreased (Schonert-Reichl & Lawlor, 2010). In a related study, Schonert-Reichl et al. (2015) followed 99 fourth and fifth grade children assigned to either a 12-lesson MindUP intervention or to the control group. Results indicated increased mindfulness abilities post-assessment for the youth in the intervention, along with significant positive effects on optimism, empathy, and perspective taking. There were marginal improvements in reaction time and math grades, as compared to the control group. Here again, teacher expectation bias may limit these findings, and further research is warranted.

Website for MindUP: https://mindup.org/

Still Quiet Place

The program Still Quiet Place (Saltzman, 2014) is a program modeled on MBSR and designed for children and adults alike, with modified language and practices for youth aged 5–18. The goal of the program is to improve behavioral and emotional self-regulation and general well-being of youth through mindfulness practices. Still Quiet Place requires the facilitator to attend either an in-person training or complete a 10-week online course. The structure of the program in the schools consists of eight weekly sessions wherein students learn mindfulness, breathwork, body scanning, and loving kindness practices. Home practice is encouraged via audio-guided meditations.

To date, no published peer-reviewed research on the Still Quiet Place school program has been conducted. However, a study of a self-referred nonclinical community sample of 24 families (31 children and 27 parents), with wait-list controls, found that those who engaged in the Still

Quiet Place curriculum had beneficial changes in attention, mood, and metacognitive domains (compassion and mindfulness; Saltzman & Goldin, 2008). Formal (e.g., guided sitting, body scan) and informal (e.g., a meaningful pause, mindfulness in daily life) practice was parsed out and analyzed separately, with informal practice showing greater improvement in depressive symptoms; formal practice explained a significant amount of variance in post-intervention cognitive control of attention, after accounting for baseline cognitive control. Though these results are encouraging, in order to fully understand the strengths and limitations of this program, peer-reviewed published research studies of Still Quiet Place are needed.

Website for Still Quiet Place: *www.stillquietplace.com*

Stressed Teens

Stressed Teens (2019) is an organization that houses various mindfulness programs for children and adults. Stressed Teens Mindfulness-Based Stress Reduction for Teens (MBSR-T) is an eight-week program for youth aged 13–18, based on MBSR. Specific activities in this program include meditation, body scan, mindful awareness, and heartfulness.

A research study examined the MBSR-T program with 102 adolescents aged 14–18 who were currently or previously under outpatient psychiatric care. Compared to control participants, the intervention group had significantly reduced anxiety, depressive, and somatic symptoms, and improved self-esteem and sleep quality. Completers of the MBSR-T program also reported significant declines in perceived stress, obsessive symptoms, and interpersonal problems relative to controls. More than 45% of the MBSR-T participants showed positive diagnostic change, particularly those previously diagnosed with a mood disorder; almost none of the control participants exhibited any change (Biegel et al., 2009). While this study is encouraging, more randomized controlled trials are necessary on the MBSR-T program in order to fully understand the effects of the intervention beyond a small outpatient population.

Website for Stressed Teens: *www.stressedteens.com*

Mindful Life Project

The mission of the Mindful Life Project (2021) is to teach mindfulness, yoga, expressive arts, and hip-hop dance to elementary and middle school students in underserved communities. This mindfulness program teaches self-awareness, impulse control, self-regulation, resiliency, and confidence to students in schools. In their summary report for the 2018–2019 school year, the website states that Mindful Life Project reached over 10,000 students a week in 22 underserved schools.

Internal research, posted on the Mindful Life Project webpage, notes that based on teacher ratings, 83% reported improvement in their students' self-awareness, 79% in student self-regulation, 77% in student ability to relate to one another, and 71% in attentional abilities (Mindful Life Project, 2019). Additionally, suspensions across schools were reported to be significantly lower at participating schools after implementing the program (Mindful Life Project, 2019). In a dissertation research study by Crockett-Chaney (2018), 42 fourth grade students participated in either the Mindful Life Project (n=30) curriculum or wait-list control group (n=12) for eight 30-minute weekly sessions. Compared to controls at post-assessment, children in the intervention group demonstrated an increase in mindfulness skills, improvement in self-regulation, and increased positive behavior in the classroom. Though these initial results are supportive of its use, it is recommended that more rigorous, peer-reviewed research be conducted on the use of the Mindful Life Project in schools.

Website for the Mindful Life Project: *http://mindfullifeproject.org*

Wellness Works in Schools

Wellness Works in Schools (2017) is a mindfulness-based program designed to use with youth aged 3–18 to develop health and wellness in the academic setting. The modules are presented in a series of 8–15 lessons, with an emphasis on teacher training and practice. Skills focus on addressing mental, emotional, physical, and social health for youth.

On the website for Wellness Works in Schools (2017), internal survey research notes that 94% of teachers stated the program helped their students to focus and pay attention and 82% of students reported that they could better regulate their behavior, including 76% showing an increased ability to manage stress and regulate their emotions. To date, no peer-reviewed research has been published. Further research on the effectiveness of this program is necessary.

Website for Wellness Works in Schools: *www.wellnessworksinschools.com*

Resilient Kids

Originally developed as an after-school program, Center for Resilience (2018) is now an adapted classroom curriculum for grades K–12. This program addresses the five core competencies as described by the Collaborative for Academic, Social and Emotional Learning (CASEL, 2019): self-awareness, self-management, relationship skills, social awareness, and responsible decision-making. A unique feature of this program is that it is designed to be taught throughout the academic year, with 32 weeks of curriculum offered in weekly or twice a week sessions. The curriculum includes practices such as breathwork, yoga, mindfulness movement, and meditation. Facilitators of the program attend a short, one-time workshop before implementation.

On the website, Center for Resilience (2018), results of an internal program evaluation are noted, touting "dramatic reductions in student and teacher stress; bullying; and behavior-related visits to the principal's office." However, no outside research or peer-reviewed published studies are available on this program. This program was included in this review due to its unique format integrating mindfulness curriculum into classrooms throughout the school year. More research must be conducted to understand the impact of this continuity for student benefit in the schools.

Website for Resilient Kids: www.centerforresilience.org/

Master Mind Academy

The Master Mind Academy (Innovation Research and Training, 2014) is a four-week, daily mindfulness education and substance abuse prevention program for elementary school-aged children, grades four and five. Daily lessons are led by a classroom teacher; each week one subtopic of mindfulness is covered, including awareness of the body, feelings, thoughts, and relationships. Homework activities, called "investigations," are encouraged for student practice. These extension assignments are designed to further student understanding of mindfulness and provide them with a wider variety of opportunities to practice their learned skills.

Parker and colleagues (2014) investigated the Master Mind Academy with two elementary schools that were randomly assigned to either the intervention group (n = 71) or the waitlist control group (n = 40). Compared to the control group, students who were taught the four-week *Master Mind* program by their regular classroom teachers showed significant improvements in executive functioning skills (for both girls and boys), reductions in aggression and social problems (for both girls and boys) and anxiety symptoms (girls only) at post-assessment. There was a marginally significant increase in self-control abilities for boys only. No significant differences were found between groups for intention to use substances, such as tobacco or alcohol. More research on this program is necessary in order to further evaluate its effects on well-being and substance use.

Website for Master Mind Academy: www.irtinc.us/Products/Master Mind/Overview.aspx

Inner Kids Program

The Inner Kids (Greenland, 2016) website offers blogs, guided practices, videos, and book excerpts, all free of charge, to help promote mindfulness practices for youth K–12 and their families. Though there is not a formal school-based program educators can implement, teachers and mental health professionals who work with youth can enroll in an online continuing education course designed to learn how to work with children in bolstering six essential life skills: Quieting, Focusing, Seeing, Reframing, Caring, and Connecting.

Though there is little peer-reviewed research specifically on the Inner Kids program, the website consists of a variety of mindfulness acceptance practices (MAPS) that have been supported in other research. There is one study conducted by Flook et al. (2010) using the MAPS specifically from the Inner Kids program. It found that the mindfulness practices introduced in the general education setting were particularly beneficial for children with executive functioning difficulties. For children who initially showed deficits in their executive functioning, participating in the Inner Kids MAPs training led to improved executive functioning skills. More quality research is needed to evaluate the effectiveness of this program.

Website for Inner Kids Program: www.susankaisergreenland.com

Learning to Breathe

Learning to Breathe (Broderick, 2013) is a school-based mindfulness curriculum created for adolescents, as well as college-age emerging adults. It is administered in classroom or group settings. The curriculum is designed to strengthen attention and emotion regulation, cultivate gratitude and compassion, increase stress management skills, and help participants integrate mindfulness into daily life. Based on MBSR, the curriculum also draws from ACT and other mindfulness-based cognitive therapies. The program contains six structured lessons but can be expanded to twelve or more sessions. Learning to Breathe has been recognized in the 2019 CASEL Guide as meeting research criteria for effective social and emotional learning programs.

There is extensive research on the Learning to Breathe curriculum, more than many other school-based mindfulness programs. Several studies have found evidence of the Learning to Breathe curriculum as being effective at decreasing anxiety and stress reactions in youth (Eva & Thayer, 2017; Metz et al., 2013). Shomaker et al. (2017) investigated the impact of the Learning to Breathe curriculum versus cognitive behavioral therapy (CBT) group therapy for teenage females at risk for depression and type 2 diabetes. At post-treatment and six-month follow up, participants in the Learning to Breathe program had greater decreases in depressive symptoms and insulin resistance, including fasting insulin, than adolescents in the CBT group. In a study by Fung et al. (2016),

19 low-income ethnic minority middle-school students participated in an eight-week intervention using the Learning to Breathe curriculum. A significant reduction in youth reported internalizing problems and parent-reported externalizing problems was found. Broderick and Metz (2009) used the Learning to Breathe curriculum with 120 female high school seniors as a part of their health curriculum. Relative to the control group, participants reported decreased tiredness, somatic complaints, and negative affect and increased feelings of self-acceptance, calmness, and relaxation. These studies provide positive empirical support for the Learning to Breathe curriculum. Replication studies, including a diversity of populations, is recommended.

Website for Learning to Breathe: https://learning2breathe.org/

How to Choose the Right Program for Your Classroom or School

With so many options, it can be challenging to decide which program is right for your student population. There are a few factors you will need to consider in any decision, including the age of your students, the level of training necessary to administer the program, the amount of time you have to allot to the program during the school day, and the intended outcome goals.

We recommend that you choose the program with the collaboration of the other professionals in your school or classroom, including, but not limited to your principal, teachers, school-based mental health providers and, if relevant, parents. The latter is particularly important if working in a family cooperative school setting. Whatever program you choose, you will need to adapt the program to meet the needs of your particular students, including their developmental level, cultural background, and cognitive functioning. Please refer to Chapter 7 for more information on adapting the materials for various student populations. See the Ready, Set, Go! Checklist (Form 6.1) to help structure your process for running a classroom or school-wide program.

Conclusion

This chapter overviewed some of the practical considerations and support for implementing classroom and school-wide mindfulness practices. A sampling of school-based mindfulness programs was reviewed. The majority of the research indicates that school-based mindfulness programs for students are useful in a variety of ways, including increasing student executive functioning and feelings of well-being, while decreasing anxiety and mood disordered symptoms. It is imperative that high-quality, experimental control group designed studies continue to assess the utility of these programs with a variety of populations.

Form 6.1

Ready-Set-Go! Checklist

CLASSROOM AND SCHOOL-WIDE PROGRAMS

Table 6.3

Task	Date Sent/Accomplished
Create Buy-In (teachers meeting, speak with principal, etc.)	
Send out Parent Letter Describing the Selected Program	
Determine Who Will Implement the Lessons (Teacher, School Psychologist, etc.)	
Determine Time/Day to Begin the Curriculum	
Review all Curriculum Sessions, Making Modifications as Necessary; Prepare Needed Materials	
Start Your Program!	

References

Bakosh, L. S., Snow, R. M., Tobias, J. M., Houlihan, J. L., & Barbosa-Leiker, C. (2014). Maximizing mindful learning: Mindful awareness intervention improves elementary school students' quarterly grades. *Mindfulness*, 7(1), 5967.

Bakosh, L. S., Tobias Mortlock, J. M., Querstret, D., & Morison, L. (2018). Audio-guided mindfulness training in schools and its effect on academic attainment: Contributing to theory and practice. *Learning and Instruction*, 58, 34–41.

Biegel, G. M., Brown, K. W., Shapiro, S. L., & Schubert, C. M. (2009). Mindfulness-based stress reduction for the treatment of adolescent psychiatric outpatients: A randomized clinical trial. *Journal of Consulting and Clinical Psychology*, 77(5), 855–866.

Black, D. S., & Fernando, R. (2014). Mindfulness training and classroom behavior among lower-income and ethnic minority elementary school children. *Journal of Child and Family Studies*, 23(7), 1242–1246.

Broderick, P. C. (2013). *Learning to Breathe: About L2B*. Learning to Breathe. https://learning2breathe.org/

Broderick, P. C., & Metz, S. (2009). Learning to BREATHE: A pilot trial of a mindfulness curriculum for adolescents. *Advances in School Mental Health Promotion*, 2(1), 35–46.

Center for Resilience. (2018). *Who we are*. www.centerforresilience.org/our-mission/

Collaborative for Academic, Social, and Emotional Learning. (2019). *CASEL program guides – Effective social and emotional learning programs*. https://casel.org/guide/

Crockett-Chaney, E. (2018). *Impact of a school-based mindfulness intervention on children's self- regulation* [Doctoral dissertation, The University of San Francisco]. USF Scholarship Repository. https://repository.usfca.edu/diss

Eva, A. L., & Thayer, N. M. (2017). Learning to BREATHE: A pilot study of a mindfulness-based intervention to support marginalized youth. *Journal of Evidence-Based Complementary & Alternative Medicine*, 22(4), 580–591.

Flook, L., Smalley, S. L., Kitil, M. J., Galla, B. M., Kaiser-Greenland, S., Locke, J., Ishijima, E., & Kasari, C. (2010). Effects of mindful awareness practices on executive functions in elementary school children. *Journal of Applied School Psychology*, 26(1), 70–95.

Fung, J., Guo, S., Jim, J., Bear, L., & Lau, A. (2016). A pilot randomized trial evaluating a school-based mindfulness intervention for ethnic minority youth. *Mindfulness*, 7(4), 819–828.

Greenland, S. K. (2016). *Inner Kids program*. www.susankaisergreenland.com

Hanson, R., & Mendius, R. (2009). *Buddha's brain: The practical neuroscience of happiness, love, and wisdom*. New Harbinger Publication.

Houlihan, J., & Bakosh, L. S. (2011). *Inner Explorer program*. Inner Explorer. https://innerexplorer.org/

Innovation Research and Training. (2014). *Master Mind Academy*. www.irtinc.us/Products/MasterMind/Overview.aspx

Kabat-Zinn, J. (2003). Mindfulness-based interventions in context: Past, present, and future. *Clinical Psychology: Science and Practice*, 10(2), 144–156.

Liehr, P., & Diaz, N. (2010). A pilot student examining the effect of mindfulness on depression and anxiety for minority children. *Archives of Psychiatric Nursing*, 24(1), 69–71.

Livheim, F., Hayes, L., Ghaderi, A., Magnusdottir, T., Högfeldt, A., Rowse, J., Turner, S., Hayes, S. C., & Tengström, A. (2014). The effectiveness of acceptance and commitment therapy for adolescent mental health: Swedish and Australian pilot outcomes. *Journal of Child and Family Studies, 24*(4), 1016–1030.

Metz, S. M., Frank, J. L., Reibel, D., Cantrell, T., Sanders, R., & Broderick, P. C. (2013). The effectiveness of the learning to BREATHE program on adolescent emotion regulation. *Research in Human Development, 10*(3), 252–272.

Mindful Life Project. (2019). *2018–2019 End of year report.* http://mindfullifeproject.org/wp-content/uploads/2019/12/final-mindful_life_project_2018-2019_report.pdf

Mindful Life Project. (2021). *Mindful life project.* www.mindfullifeproject.org/

Mindful Schools. (2015a). *Mindfulness fundamentals.* www.mindfulschools.org/training/mindfulness-fundamentals/

Mindful Schools. (2015b). *Research on mindfulness.* www.mindfulschools.org/about-mindfulness/research/

MindUP. (2003). *A program for empowering children through mindful practice based in neuroscience.* https://mindup.org/

National Center for Complementary and Integrative Medicine. (2017). *Meditation: In depth.* NCCIH. www.nccih.nih.gov/health/meditation-in-depth

Parker, A. E., Kupersmidt, J. B., Mathis, E. T., Scull, T. M., & Sims, C. (2014). The impact of mindfulness education on elementary school students: Evaluation of the Master Mind program. *Advances in School Mental Health Promotion, 7*(3), 184–204.

Roodenrys, S., Badawi, A., & Lovegrove, W. (2017). How strong is the evidence that mindfulness produces healthy psychological changes in children? In T. Ditrich, R. Wiles, & B. Lovegrove (Eds.), *Mindfulness and education: Research and practice* (pp. 33–54). Cambridge Scholars Publishing.

Saltzman, A. (2014). *A still quiet place: A mindfulness program for teaching children and adolescents to ease stress and difficult emotions.* New Harbinger Publications.

Saltzman, A., & Goldin, P. (2008). Mindfulness-based stress reduction for school-age children. In L. A. Greco & S. C. Hayes (Eds.), *Acceptance and mindfulness treatments for children and adolescents: A practitioner's guide* (pp. 139–161). New Harbinger Publications.

Schonert-Reichl, K. A., & Lawlor, M. S. (2010). The effects of a mindfulness-based education program on pre- and early adolescents' well-being and social and emotional competence. *Mindfulness, 1*(3), 137–151.

Schonert-Reichl, K. A., Oberle, E, Lawlor, M. S., Abbot, D., Thomson, K., Oberlander, T., & Diamond, A. (2015). Enhancing cognitive and social-emotional development through a simple-to-administer mindfulness-based school program for elementary school children: A randomized controlled trial. *Developmental Psychology, 51*(1), 52–66.

Shomaker, L. B., Bruggink, S., Pivarunas, P., Skoranski, A., Foss, J., Chaffin, E., Dalager, S., Annameier, S., Quaglia, J., Brown, K. W., Broderick, P., & Bell, C. (2017). Pilot randomized controlled trial of a mindfulness-based group in adolescent girls at risk for type 2 diabetes with depressive symptoms. *Complementary Therapies in Medicine, 32*, 66–74.

Sofer, O. J. (2016). *Heartfulness practice.* Mindful Schools. www.mindfulschools.org/personal-practice/heartfulness-practice/

Stressed Teens. (2019). *Stressed teens.* www.stressedteens.com

Szabo, T., & Dixon, M. (2016). Contextual behavioural science and education. In R. Zettle, S. Hayes, D. Barnes-Holmes, & A. Biglan (Eds.), *The Wiley handbook of contextual behavioural science.* John Wiley & Sons.

Wellness Works in Schools. (2017). *About wellness works in schools.* Kinder Associates. www.wellnessworksinschools.com

7 Creating Systemic Change and Adapting Practices for Different Populations

Roadmap to Chapter 7:

This chapter overviews ideas for how to successfully engage schools in adopting mindfulness and acceptance-based programs and how to adapt practices for different populations. Specifically, it covers:

- creating systemic change within the school setting
- using mindfulness and acceptance practices for youth with developmental or social impairments
- cultural considerations for the use of mindfulness in the schools
- frequently asked questions (FAQs) when introducing mindfulness and acceptance practices to stakeholders

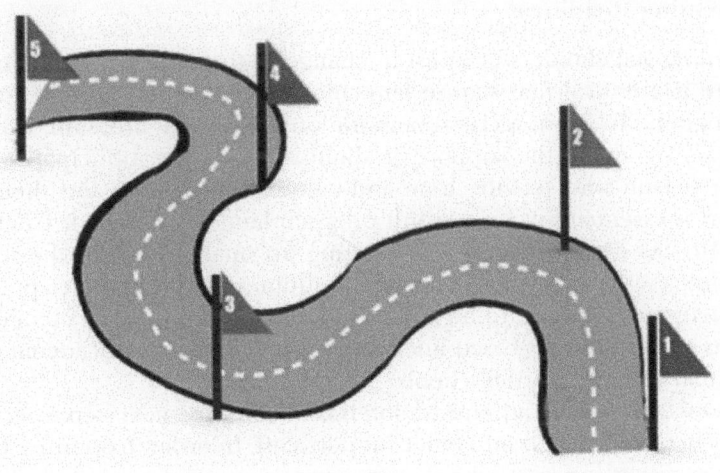

DOI: 10.4324/9781003318101-7

As described in Chapter 2, research supports mindfulness and acceptance practices as effective tools for youth with a variety of presenting concerns. This chapter first discusses how to create initial buy-in and longer-term sustainability for using these practices as prevention and intervention tools. The chapter then discusses adapting the materials to work with various populations.

Securing the School Community's Buy-In

Before introducing mindfulness and acceptance practices into your work with youth in the schools, it is important to create buy-in with those with whom you will be working. Sharing the research in a digestible format with the school and parents can be a good start. Highlight how the proposed interventions can positively impact a student's emotional and social well-being, as well as their educational performance. Also consider the organizational dynamics of the school and employ strategies that will help to foster the implementation and continuation of the practices. These strategies range from examining factors that lead to optimal program buy-in to barriers that may be present in implementing a classroom or school-wide mindfulness and acceptance program.

According to Adelman and Taylor (2007) there are four critical stages of creating systemic change within schools: creating readiness, initial implementation, institutionalization, and ongoing evolution and creative renewal. Each of these overlapping phases will be explored next as they relate to launching a mindfulness program.

Creating Readiness

Getting stakeholders to invest in change in their school climate or culture is a critical first step in launching a mindfulness and acceptance program. To begin a classroom-wide or school-wide program, it is necessary to secure the support of administrators. The principal is often the person who sets the tone and culture of a school, and their support is essential for a successful program launch (Merrell & Gueldner, 2010). As described earlier for setting up small groups in the school, share research-related benefits of mindfulness and acceptance practices system-wide. Be sure to highlight information about the academic benefits of mindfulness-based intervention since impact on academics is of primary concern in the schools.

Once the school administration is on board, the next step is securing buy-in from teachers and other support staff. In order to optimize buy-in when discussing with school staff, it can be helpful to identify the collective values of the school staff and how these programs can positively contribute to a shared vision of the community they hope to build in their school. For example, if school staff identify "responsibility" as a core value, you can highlight how mindfulness and acceptance-based programs can positively contribute toward developing a school culture that promotes this value. At a staff meeting or similar venue, give a short in-service training on mindfulness and acceptance, highlighting the benefits of these practices in the schools (Adelman & Taylor, 2007). When teachers and other school staff understand the goals of a mindfulness program, it can increase their willingness to use the practices (Dariotis et al., 2017). At these meetings, questions may be asked about the use of mindfulness in the schools. As a quick reference, answers to common questions can be found on the Frequently Asked Questions (FAQ's) handout (Form 7.1).

Helping to instill a personal enthusiasm in teachers for mindfulness practices can increase their motivation for using the skills with students. Mischenko and Jennings (2019) noted that teachers' feeling passionate toward the use of mindfulness is critical. To foster this, engage teachers in their own practice of mindfulness. Practitioner use of the skills increases their passion for using it with others (Jennings, 2015). When a teacher's sense of well-being is increased, it will begin to translate into an environment of wellness for their classroom (Rechtschaffen, 2016). Additionally, involve teachers in mindfulness program selection and provide them with options of how mindfulness practices can be integrated into their classrooms. These are favorable conditions for initial teacher buy-in (Mischenko & Jennings, 2019).

Sending teachers and other school staff who will be involved in the execution of the program to a professional development program on mindfulness can be a good way to secure buy-in and increase fidelity of implementation. These trainings also rest on the principle that the teaching of mindfulness can only truly be transmitted through a practitioner who has experience with the practice themselves (Rechtschaffen, 2016). In one study, all teachers surveyed in the sample expressed willingness to attend mindfulness training if the principal could integrate it within existing meetings (Dariotis et al., 2017). Another idea could be to have a "book club" where teachers and staff are given a book on mindfulness practices, or perhaps given a link to watch a short film on mindfulness, and to have a scheduled discussion group about the content. Some ideas for books could include *Buddha's Brain: The Practical Neuroscience of Happiness, Love, and Wisdom* by Hanson and Mendius (2009) or *The Mindful Path to Self-Compassion: Freeing Yourself from Destructive Thoughts and Emotions* by Germer (2009). Educators and other stakeholders could also view the video offered by Mindful Schools (2015c), *Healthy Habits of Mind – The Science of Compassion*. This can open up discussion on the topic of the benefits of mindfulness and how to apply the practices in the schools (available at: www.mindfulschools.org/video/healthy-habits-mind/). Some programs, as discussed later in this chapter, require more formalized training for users.

Initial Implementation

During the implementation phase, program logistics, such as the physical environment where the practice will be carried out and the time of day the program will be held, will need to be determined in a way to maximize teacher support. The environment should be as free from interruption and distraction as possible, while the time of day should not pose a barrier to the program being run. Although constraints may limit when a program can be offered, scheduling merits careful consideration, as it is closely tied to student motivation and program participation. Options to consider, when feasible, include incorporating mindfulness training into physical or health education curriculum (Dariotis et al., 2017) or during existing social and emotional learning (SEL) curriculum time (Rechtschaffen, 2016).

Mindfulness program implementation should be carried out in stages, with guidance and support from an individual or organization that can help structure the execution with fidelity (Adelman & Taylor, 2007). It is important to create a clear and realistic timeline for rolling out the program, as well as clearly communicating this to administrators, teachers, and school staff, as this will help enhance stakeholder buy-in. When not using an outside organization for push-in services, it would be best if someone familiar with the program is easily accessible to teachers and staff for any questions as the program is being launched. Individuals who have experience with the program could be identified as coaches or mentors to those who are new to the school-based mindfulness program (Merrell & Gueldner, 2010).

To monitor efficacy, set up and begin some form of evaluation or assessment of the program, as further described in Chapter 9. Collect baseline data to start. Ongoing data collection can be used for both monitoring of students' progress and overall program effectiveness.

Institutionalization

In this phase of implementation, emphasis is placed on maintaining and enhancing the mindfulness program to make it a part of the fabric of the school, as opposed to a one-time event. If new programs are introduced but not institutionalized as part of the on-going culture, they fade away over time (Merrell & Gueldner, 2010). The goal in this phase is to create an identity around the use of mindfulness for the school, where teachers, staff, and administrators all experience ownership of the mindfulness practices (Adelman & Taylor, 2007). Don't limit the practice of mindfulness to those days that the program is run. Some ideas for this generalization of practices are offered later in this chapter.

Ongoing Evaluation and Creative Renewal

This phase uses mechanisms to improve the quality of the mindfulness program at the school and to enable stakeholders to continuously find ways of supporting and renewing their energy and enthusiasm regarding the program (Adelman & Taylor, 2007). Over time, users may become loose with treatment fidelity, feel over-taxed with other duties, no longer put a priority on the mindfulness practices, or forget to use the practices. Ongoing evaluation and providing feedback around the execution of the program can be critical here in order to ensure fidelity of the practices. Finding ways to invigorate school professionals around the continued use of the materials and practices is a key component to the program's long-term success (Merrell & Gueldner, 2010). As mentioned previously, integrating mindfulness into existing school structures for social emotional learning can provide continuing support for a mindfulness program (Rechtschaffen, 2016). Reviewing practices and introducing fresh ideas for implementation at faculty meetings can help keep an energized momentum for the program. Finally, consider collaborating with school administrators on how to incentivize school staff to implement these programs with fidelity, as this can be helpful in creating long-term sustainability.

Enlisting Family and Community Support

Ideally, when beginning any program at a school, consider how to have the skills being taught reinforced in and generalized to other settings. Family and other community member support for the program can be key to ensuring the use of practices outside of the school day (Rechtschaffen, 2016). The spectrum of involvement can range from simple communications sent home or posted on the school's webpage, to inviting families and other school partners to attend a training where mindfulness and acceptance practices are overviewed and the benefits to students are highlighted. As discussed in Chapter 8, mindful and compassionate parenting techniques can be offered to families to cultivate healthy environments in the home. The level of engagement offered may depend on the school's culture and the community where the mindfulness practices are being introduced. Some communities may be more resistant to mental health promotion and primary intervention activities and, therefore, more engagement efforts will be necessary so that the program is not undermined or derailed in some way (Merrell & Gueldner, 2010). Enlisting the help of influential community members, including religious leaders when appropriate, can be useful in persuading the community to have an open mind around the practices being taught. Linking mindfulness with social action, health, and well-being can help with reaching wider acceptance of the practices (Arthurson, 2017). Further discussion on culture and diversity regarding mindfulness practice is offered later in this chapter. In general, often simply getting the word out via written materials sent home or through a series of parent informational meetings held at convenient times for families to attend can be a positive and constructive way to garner support and alleviate parental concerns around new programs in the schools (Merrell & Gueldner, 2010).

The next section covers how to use mindfulness with students who have cognitive or social impairments.

Adaptation for Students with Cognitive or Social Impairments

In meeting the needs of all students in our pluralistic society, it is important to understand how to best adapt interventions for children who have cognitive delays (e.g., intellectual disabilities; ID) or social challenges (e.g., autism spectrum disorder; ASD). Though most mindfulness and acceptance-based interventions do not include such adaptations, this section will overview some considerations when working with these populations.

For youth with cognitive impairments, it is important to ensure that the materials used consider their current level of functioning. Children with cognitive delays typically acquire and process information at a slower rate, necessitating the use of repetition and a slower rate of instructional delivery (Merrell & Gueldner, 2010). Consequently, a formal mindfulness program will likely take more sessions and instructional tactics that integrate mindfulness throughout the curriculum to ensure the greatest benefit. Opportunities to practice skills with the youth throughout the day can help with their skills acquisition and generalizability of the skills. Additionally, youth with cognitive impairments or speech and language delays may have challenges processing verbal or written materials and respond better to tactile and visual stimuli (Jaime & Knowlton, 2007). Experiential activities, such as repetition of mindful breathing techniques or body scans, are typically more effective than cognitive approaches, such as cognitive defusion.

Though there must be some modification in using mindfulness and acceptance-based approaches with youth with ID, ACT-based strategies have been found to reduce the high levels of work-related stress experienced by school staff as a result of managing challenging behaviors exhibited by individuals with ID. In one study, when staff themselves used ACT, post-intervention staff in the mindfulness and acceptance group reported significantly greater reductions in distress than the control group, with these reductions maintained at 6-week follow up. The effect of the intervention was more pronounced amongst a subsample of staff that had shown higher levels of psychological distress at baseline (McConachie et al., 2014).

Youth with social impairments or ASD symptoms may also have challenges with traditional mindfulness or acceptance-based interventions and may need modifications. In general, youth with ASD have deficits in social and communication skills, including challenges identifying their feelings, in conjunction with bodily sensations (Merrell & Gueldner, 2010). Youth with ASD may think in more literal terms, so use of the many ACT metaphors might be particularly challenging (Mashal & Kasirer, 2011). Instead, use of direct skills instruction and modeling, such as in 4x8 breathing, use of visuals, and engaging youth in concrete exercises oftentimes used with younger individuals can assist in skills acquisition (Arthur-Kelly et al., 2009; Feldman, 2019).

With these recommended modifications, children with ASD symptoms have been found to benefit from mindfulness-based interventions. In a study by de Bruin and colleagues (2014), adolescents with ASD reported an increase in quality of life and a decrease in ruminative thoughts after intervention. Additionally, although parents reported no improvement in their teens' specific ASD core symptoms, they did report their teens as having improved social communication and responsiveness and decreased cognitive rumination. Parents who also themselves participated in the program reported improved competence in parenting and increased mindfulness. Other studies have concurred with these findings, with improvement in youth emotional regulation and adaptive skills after mindfulness intervention, along with increased mindfulness for parent participants (Salem-Guirgis et al., 2019). Therefore, mindfulness and acceptance-based interventions do hold some promise for children with ASD, with appropriate modifications.

Cultural Considerations in Mindfulness, Acceptance, and Yoga Practices

Through its programs, schools must have cultural sensitivity and respect for the practices of the families they serve (Jennings, 2015). Practitioners should strive to be interculturally effective when working with their target population and knowledgeable of various aspects of their participating community's culture, including different religious practices, ethnic backgrounds, acculturation levels, immigration histories, and so on.

Mindfulness has been criticized by some due to its association with religion, mainly Buddhism (Agger, 2015). This has become less pronounced over the last decade as mindfulness has become more mainstream, however, practitioners should keep this in mind, especially when working with conservative religious communities. Though mindfulness is used as a path toward insight in the Buddhist tradition, the practice is not in-and-of-itself religious. John Kabat-Zinn originally refined

Table 7.1 Key distinctions between Buddhism, mindfulness, and ACT.

Practice	Basis	Idea of the Self	Religious?
Buddhism	Dharma teachings/ Religious: not directed at mental health, but rather enlightenment	See through the delusions of self for goal of enlightenment	Yes
Mindfulness	Increase present moment awareness	Increase present moment awareness of the self	No
ACT	Increase psychological flexibility	Reinforces the sense of an enduring self, or self-as-context	No

mindfulness practice for use in a secular medical setting when he developed MBSR in 1979 (Kabat-Zinn, 2013). Mindfulness, as used in mental health, is also a secular practice. The religious practice of Buddhism parts ways with the Westernized use of mindfulness, with the two being very distinct. ACT, which includes mindfulness, also differs from Buddhist practices in various ways. Table 7.1 can be used as a quick guide to these concepts.

For the school setting, it is often most appropriate to emphasize the secular practice of mindfulness. However, restoring or adding cultural context into mindfulness practices may help some groups, such as recent immigrants from Asia, feel more comfortable with the intervention and draw strength from their own background (Agger, 2015; Kirmayer, 2015).

Some have also argued that using mindfulness and yoga with youth should include recognition of the cultural roots of the practice and awareness of the cultural background of the participants (Hagen & Nayar, 2014). A brief history of mindfulness and yoga, as offered next, can help illuminate its use in Western society and increase cultural sensitivity toward the practice. Mindfulness is a practice that people have been using for thousands of years and is integrated into various religious and secular traditions – from Hinduism and Buddhism to yoga and, more recently, non-religious meditation. In general, mindfulness was popularized in the East by religious institutions and spiritual practices, while in the West its popularity can be traced to particular people, such as Jon Kabat-Zinn (Kabat-Zinn, 2013), and secular institutions. However, even the secular tradition of mindfulness in the West owes its roots to Eastern practices (Selva, 2022). Yoga originated in India between 200 BC and 200 AD, as an ancient spiritual practice of self-realization. However, the British saw it as threatening during their colonization of India and they banned it beginning in the 1700s and lasting until the mid-1900s. Today, there is conversation around the "cultural appropriation" of mindfulness and yoga. Cultural appropriation is the taking, marketing, and glamorizing of cultural practices from historically oppressed populations (Askegaard & Eckhardt, 2012; Gandhi & Wolff, 2017).

The question of whether one is appreciating versus appropriating the cultural practices of yoga and mindfulness is complex. Are yoga and mindfulness sterilized by removing evidence of their Eastern roots so that they don't "offend" Westerner practitioners? On the other hand, are the practices glamorized through commercialism and consumerism, such as tattoos in Sanskrit, the loose use of the word "namaste," and T-shirts sporting Hindu deities or the word "Om"? Most practitioners do not learn about Hindu tradition or Indian cultural history, instead primarily focusing on the health and fitness aspects of the practice. Therefore, it is argued that these practitioners are perpetuating the cultural appropriation of mindfulness and yoga by diluting its true meaning and depth (Askegaard & Eckhardt, 2012; Gandhi & Wolff, 2017). Gandhi and Wolff (2017) argue that this modern-day cultural appropriation of these practices is a continuation of power inequity, maintaining the pattern of Westerners consuming the "stuff of culture" that is trendy, while ignoring honoring the origin culture (arguably something that we strive to not do in an academic setting, such as schools).

Given this, what is the recommendation for how we can best approach yoga and mindfulness practices in Western schools? Gandhi and Wolff (2017) recommend practitioners take a series of steps, some of which are relevant in the school setting. First, they recommend practitioners have some awareness of the roots of the practice they are using and give humility, respect, and reverence toward the originating culture (Gandhi & Wolff, 2017). In the schools, giving basic context as to the history and origin of mindfulness and yoga practices to students could be incorporated into the sessions, as overviewed earlier in this section. Next, they recommend practitioners create space for conversations about cultural appropriation and cultural accountability with the users of their services. Additionally, they encourage eliminating any barriers to access (Gandhi & Wolff, 2017), such as encouraging yoga studios to offer reduced rates or no-cost practices to students at local primary and secondary schools.

In summary, it is recommended that because Eastern and Western use of mindfulness-based practices are framed by significantly different systems of meaning, the practitioner must consider the background of those they are serving to assist the cultural adaptation and application of the intervention (Agger, 2015). Treatment practices cannot be transposed wholly from one cultural setting to another, but instead require consideration of the cultural background of the student (Kirmayer, 2015). Additionally, honoring the origin of the practices of mindfulness in the various ways explored in this section does not have to conflict with the Western use of the practices.

Conclusion

As mindfulness and acceptance practices are becoming more widely used in the school setting, consider best practices regarding implementation of these techniques, including creating systemic change in the school setting and adapting interventions for various populations. This chapter overviewed some of the ways of enlisting stakeholders and modifying the practices for developmental, social, and cultural differences. Given the ever-changing landscape of mental health in the school setting, it is important to remain current on the latest recommendations for best practices in the setting where you wish to implement these interventions.

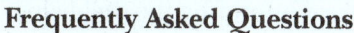

Form 7.1

Frequently Asked Questions

What is mindfulness?

Mindfulness is paying attention in a nonjudgmental way to the present moment.

What is acceptance as it relates to acceptance practices?

Acceptance is intentionally moving toward present-moment experiences, even those considered uncomfortable or painful, rather than attempting to avoid or change them.

Who can benefit from these practices?

Preschool-aged children to adults can benefit from mindfulness practices, whereas middle-elementary aged children to adults can benefit from both mindfulness and acceptance practices.

What if there is no time to implement mindfulness practices?

Mindfulness practices can be integrated into your life without designating blocks of time to practice. For example, mindfulness can be applied to eating, walking, and other common life activities. Mindfulness has also been shown to be helpful as an integrated classroom-wide practice, such as taking in deep breaths before test taking or using mindful listening during transitions in the school day.

What are the benefits of mindfulness and acceptance practices?

There are many benefits to using mindfulness and acceptance practices, including reduced stress and anxiety, improved immune functioning, improved emotional states and regulation, increased focus, and increased overall mental well-being.

Is mindfulness religious?

No, mindfulness is not religious, it is simply paying attention to the present moment.

How is mindfulness different from relaxation?

The intention behind mindfulness is different from that of relaxing. In mindfulness, the intention is to have nonjudgmental awareness of the present moment. When relaxing, the intention is to become relaxed, which can encompass a wide range of activities, such as lying in bed, watching television, playing tennis, and so on (not necessarily in a mindful way).

Are there risks involved in mindfulness?

Mindfulness is a safe and non-invasive tool for improving the well-being of a wide-range of groups. However, it is always important to pay attention to your own experiences when practicing mindfulness and make adjustments, if needed.

References

Adelman, H. S., & Taylor, L. (2007). Systemic change for school improvement. *Journal of Educational and Psychological Consultation, 17*(1), 55–77.

Agger, I. (2015). Calming the mind: Healing after mass atrocity in Cambodia. *Transcultural Psychiatry, 52*(4), 543–560.

Arthur-Kelly, M., Sigafoos, J., Green, V., Mathisen, B., & Arthur-Kelly, R. (2009). Issues in the use of visual supports to promote communication in individuals with autism spectrum disorder. *Disability and Rehabilitation, 31*(18), 1474–1486.

Arthurson, K. (2017). Mindfulness stripped bare: Some critical reflections from the mindfulness at school evaluation. In T. Ditrich, R. Wiles, & B. Lovegrove (Eds.), *Mindfulness and education: Research and practice* (pp. 33–54). Cambridge Scholars Publishing.

Askegaard, S., & Eckhardt, G. M. (2012). Global yoga: Re-appropriation in the Indian consumptionscape. *Marketing Theory, 12*(1), 45–60.

Dariotis, J. K., Mirabal-Beltran, R., Cluxton-Keller, F., Gould, L. F., Greenberg, M. T., & Mendelson, T. (2017). A qualitative exploration of implementation factors in a school-based mindfulness and yoga program: Lessons learned from students and teachers. *Psychology in the Schools, 54*(1), 53–69.

de Bruin, E. I., Zijlstra, B. J., & Bögels, S. M. (2014). The meaning of mindfulness in children and adolescents: Further validation of the child and adolescent mindfulness measure (CAMM) in two independent samples from the Netherlands. *Mindfulness, 5*(4), 422–430.

Feldman, H. M. (2019). How young children learn language and speech. *Pediatrics Review, 40*(8), 398–411.

Gandhi, S., & Wolff, L. (2017). *Yoga and the roots of cultural appropriation.* Praxis Center. www.kzoo.edu/praxis/yoga/

Germer, C. (2009). *The mindful path to self-compassion: Freeing yourself from destructive thoughts and emotions.* Guilford Press.

Hagen, I., & Nayar, U. S. (2014). Yoga for children and young people's mental health and well-being: Research review and reflections on the mental health potentials of yoga. *Frontiers in Psychiatry, 5*, 35.

Hanson, R., & Mendius, R. (2009). *Buddha's brain: The practical neuroscience of happiness, love, and wisdom.* New Harbinger Publication.

Jaime, K., & Knowlton, E. (2007). Visual supports for students with behavior and cognitive challenges. *Intervention in School and Clinic, 42*(5), 259–270.

Jennings, P. A. (2015). *Mindfulness for teachers: Simple skills for peace and productivity in the classroom (the Norton series on the social neuroscience of education).* W.W. Norton & Company.

Kabat-Zinn, J. (2013). *Full Catastrophe Living: Using the Wisdom of Your Body and Mind to Face Stress, Pain, and Illness.* Bantam Dell.

Kirmayer, L. J. (2015). Mindfulness in cultural context. *Transcultural Psychiatry, 52*(4), 447–469.

Mashal, N., & Kasirer, A. (2011). Thinking maps enhance metaphoric competence in children with autism and learning disabilities. *Research in Developmental Disabilities, 32*(6), 2045–2054.

McConachie, D. A. J., McKenzie, K., Morris, P. G., & Walley, R. M. (2014). Acceptance and mindfulness-based stress management for support staff caring for individuals with intellectual disabilities. *Research in Developmental Disabilities,* *35*(6), 1216–1227.

Merrell, K. W., & Gueldner, B. A. (2010). *The Guilford practical intervention in the schools series. Social and emotional learning in the classroom: Promoting mental health and academic success.* Guilford Press.

Mindful Schools. (2015c). *Healthy habits of mind – The science of compassion.* www. mindfulschools.org/video/healthy-habits-mind/

Mischenko, P. P., & Jennings, P. A. (2019). Cultivating passion for practicing and teaching mindfulness: A multiple-case study of compassionate schools project teachers. In P. A. Jennings (Ed.), *The mindful school: Transforming school culture through mindfulness and compassion* (pp. 135–165). Guilford Press.

Rechtschaffen, D. (2016). *The mindful education workbook: Lessons for teaching mindfulness to students.* W.W. Norton & Company.

Salem-Guirgis, S., Albaum, C., Tablon, P., Riosa, P. B., Nicholas, D. B., Drmic, I. E., & Weiss, J. A. (2019). MYmind: A concurrent group-based mindfulness intervention for youth with autism and their parents. *Mindfulness, 10*(9), 1730–1743.

Selva, J. (2022). History of mindfulness from East to West and religion to science. *Positive Psychology.* https://positivepsychology.com/history-of-mindfulness/

8 Mindfulness and ACT Techniques for Adult Stakeholders

Roadmap to Chapter 8:

This chapter explores the use of mindfulness and acceptance techniques for adult stakeholders. Specifically, it will cover the following:

- mindfulness and ACT techniques for use with teachers, parents, and other caregivers
- an overview of specific programs and apps for use with caregivers and educators
- teacher burnout and compassion fatigue

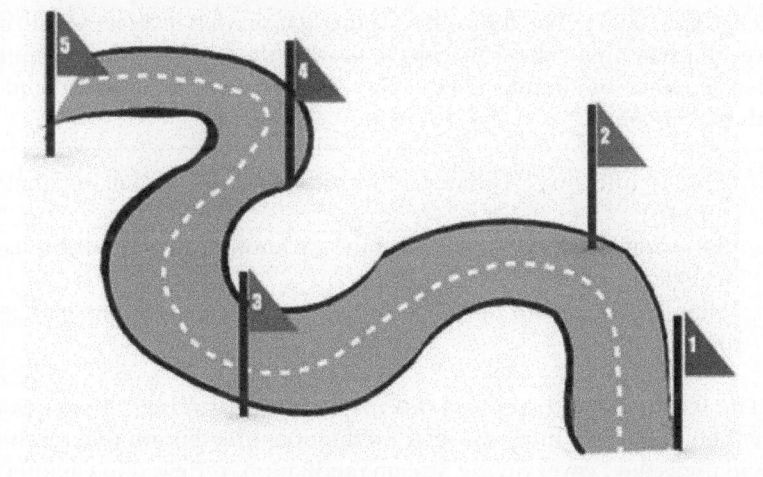

In addition to students, school personnel can benefit from mindfulness practices, from helping with classroom management to educator self-care. Stress, burnout, and compassion fatigue are common experiences for those working in the school setting, including teachers,

DOI: 10.4324/9781003318101-8

administrators, and school- related mental health professionals. Mindfulness and acceptance practices can address some of these concerns. Mindfulness and ACT techniques have also been successfully used with parents as a part of parenting-based intervention.

Mindfulness for Teachers and Other School Professionals

Mindfulness interventions have been found to reduce teachers' stress levels and improve their relations with students (Emerson et al., 2017; Taylor et al., 2016). Teachers who bring mindfulness into their classrooms find personal benefits, as well as in classroom management, and improved academics for their students.

Mindfulness techniques for adults are similar to those used with children. Breathwork, meditation, yoga, and heartfulness exercises are all common components of mindfulness programs for teachers. Reviewing the research behind the use of mindfulness for teachers and in the classroom can prove helpful for those new to the practice. As with children, breathwork, such as 4x8 breathing, is recommended as an initial technique on which to focus (see Chapter 3.)

Meditation and use of mantras can be helpful for teachers in their mindfulness practices. Common to many mantras is acknowledgment of a challenge or painful circumstance, identifying shared humanity around the experience, then completing with a compassionate statement (Ackerman, 2017). The following is a meditation that involves vocalizing three self-statements that can assist in moving the teacher toward a mindful acceptance of circumstances. These mantras are best used coupled with 4x8 breaths.

1. "This is suffering" (whatever the teacher is experiencing that is painful);
2. "Suffering is part of being human" (acknowledge that all humans struggle and suffer);
3. "May I care about and support myself" (a self-compassionate phrase).

The teacher silently repeats this mantra in their minds as they practice their deep breathing. Another meditation intervention that teachers could use is the Leaves on the Stream meditation, reviewed in Chapter 5.

Yoga has been successfully used with teachers to improve mental well-being. Yoga-based programs have been found to increase teachers' positive affect, distress tolerance, and improve physical well-being, such as decreasing blood pressure and cortisol response (Harris et al., 2016). Yoga has also been found to reduce stress and burnout for other school-based employees (Harris et al., 2016; Nosaka & Okamura, 2015). Using the poses described in Chapter 3, consider training school staff in basic yoga stretches. Additionally, a yoga instructor could make a visit during a staff meeting to engage them in a few simple poses. Staff can begin to incorporate these into their day. A teacher in-service training program focused on a yoga regimen could also be offered during a non-instructional workday. Some yoga studios offer discounts for teaching professionals or will offer group rates for schools. Heartfulness activities have been found beneficial for teachers in producing positive mood, buffering stress and burnout, and increasing compassion for themselves and their students (Emmons & McCullough, 2003; Klimecki et al., 2013). A relatively simple heartfulness activity that can be used with adults is gratitude journaling. A couple of nights each week before bed, the teacher writes down one thing they are grateful for that day. First thing the next morning, the teacher reads the positive note to themselves to begin their day with a grateful outlook. Another activity involves the teacher writing a letter to themselves from the perspective of a compassionate friend. First, the teacher thinks about the imperfections and insecurities that make them feel anxious or inadequate, taking note of the emotions that come up around those thoughts. Second, they write a supportive letter to themselves from the perspective of an unconditionally loving imaginary friend. This friend knows about the teacher's feelings of insecurity and inadequacies, but also knows all about the teacher's gifts and strengths. The final step is for the teacher to read the letter, perhaps a day later with some distance from it. The key is to let the words sink in from this unconditionally loving friend so that the "friend's" compassion becomes their own self-compassion (Ackerman, 2017). Teachers could also consider joining a local yoga studio, mindfulness, or meditation group, or engage in self-study with books (e.g., *Burnout and Trauma Related Employment Stress: Acceptance and Commitment Strategies in the Helping Professions* by Holland et al., 2021) and webinars geared toward the practice of mindfulness. There are also some mindfulness programs and phone apps that are specifically geared toward educators, which are overviewed in the next section.

Structured Mindfulness Programs for Teachers

In addition to the school-wide mindfulness programs reviewed in Chapter 6, there are group adult mindfulness programs that have been specially designed for educators in the K–12 system. Four such programs are overviewed in Table 8.1, with more detailed descriptions to follow.

Cultivating Awareness and Resilience in Education (CARE). The CARE program (Garrison Institute, 2019) introduces basic mindfulness activities (e.g., short periods of silent reflection) and progresses to how to bring mindfulness to challenging situations teachers often encounter during their school day. Emotional skills instruction in the CARE

Table 8.1 Mindfulness programs for educators.

Name	Length	Description	Outcomes
Cultivating Awareness and Resilience in Education (CARE) (Garrison Institute, 2019)	4, day-long sessions over 4–5 weeks. [a]	Incorporates basic and applied mindfulness activities in an educational setting, emotional skills instruction, and caring practice and mindful listening.	Jennings et al. (2017) found that in a sample of 224 teachers, participants reported increases in mindfulness and emotional regulation, decreases in psychological distress, and higher observed classroom productivity compared to controls.
Brown MBSR for K–12 Educators (MBSR; Brown School of Public Health, 2019)	37 hours. Optional 8-hour instructor certification available. [a]	Educators learn and apply mindfulness techniques through instruction, interactive activities, journaling, and developing a mindfulness support plan to implement in their classrooms.	No peer-reviewed research has been conducted examining the efficacy of the Brown program; however, substantial evidence exists supporting the use of MBSR.
Stress Management and Relaxation Techniques in Education (SMART) (Passage Works, 2014)	20 hours of coursework, once a week for 8 weeks after school, followed by a half-day retreat.	Helps educators reconnect to professional meaning and purpose, find balance, cultivate their emotional intelligence, and improve their well-being.	Roeser et al. (2013) found that in a sample of 113 K–12 teachers, participants compared to waitlist controls reported decreased anxiety, depression, and burnout, and increased attention, mindfulness, working memory capacity, and self-compassion.
Mindfulness Based Wellness Education (MWBE).	2.5-hour long course once per week for 8 weeks.	Largely targets pre-service teachers and focuses on teaching mindfulness to promote health and prevent the development of stress-related problems.	Poulin (2009) examined two groups of pre-service teachers and found that participants showed improvements in mindfulness, health, and feelings of teaching efficacy compared to controls.

a Summer intensive formats available.

curriculum promotes understanding, recognition, and regulation of emotion. The CARE program also promotes empathy and compassion through caring practice and mindful listening activities. The program is designed to be presented in one of two formats to educators: four day-long sessions spread out over four to five weeks, or through a five-day annual summer retreat at the Garrison Institute. Intersession coaching via phone and internet supports the practice and application of the teachers' new mindfulness skills.

The website for the Garrison Institute (2019) notes that research has consistently found that CARE significantly improves well-being and reduces stress among teacher participants. In a large randomized controlled trial of the CARE program, 224 teachers completed 30 hours of in-person training, in addition to inter-session phone coaching. Teachers completed self-report measures and assessments of their participating students (over 5,000) before and after the intervention. Teachers' classrooms were observed and coded using the Classroom Assessment Scoring System (CLASS). Teachers in the intervention had statistically significant increases in mindfulness and adaptive emotion regulation and lowered psychological distress. Additionally, CARE classrooms demonstrated higher degrees of productivity than controls (Jennings et al., 2017).

Brown MBSR for K–12 Educators. The 37-hour MBSR for K–12 Educators course (Brown School of Public Health, 2019) is a professional development opportunity for teachers to personally immerse themselves in mindfulness on both an academic and an experiential level. It also addresses how to bring mindfulness to their students. Teachers who complete the MBSR for K–12 Educators course can opt to receive eight additional hours of training to prepare them to become a mindfulness leader within the school. The Summer Intensive is another training option. It is an initial online course for teachers consisting of eight hours of introduction to mindfulness practice before four days of in-person class time. The first three days of the in-person segment are devoted to personal practice and understanding how to share mindfulness with students through didactic teaching, interactive activities, and journaling. The fourth day is focused on teachers developing a mindfulness support plan in their classrooms. No peer-reviewed research specific to the Brown program is available, though its foundation of MBSR is well-supported.

Stress Management and Relaxation Techniques in Education (SMART). SMART in Education (Passage Works, 2014) is an evidenced-based personal practice program designed especially for faculty and staff working in K–12 settings. The mission of the SMART program is to help teachers reconnect to personal and professional meaning and purpose, to find balance and cultivate their emotional intelligence, and to improve their mental and physical well-being. The program is 20 hours in length and delivered once a week for eight weeks after school, along with a half day retreat. Currently this program is only being offered in Colorado, though has been piloted in other states. In a randomized, waitlist control study by Roeser et al. (2013), 113 elementary and secondary school teachers who completed the program reported decreased anxiety, depression, and burnout, and increased attention, mindfulness, working memory capacity, and levels of self-compassion.

Mindfulness-Based Wellness Education. The Mindfulness-Based Wellness Education (MBWE) program is a mindfulness training targeting helping professions, namely pre-service teachers. The eight-week course teaches mindfulness practices to aid in health promotion and intervention for individuals at risk for developing stress-related problems, such as those going into education as a career.

In a study by Poulin (2009), two groups of teacher trainees completed MBWE as part of an elective course focusing on stress and burnout. MBWE participants experienced improvements in mindfulness, health, and feelings of teaching efficacy, in comparison to the control group, who completed other optional courses. In one intervention group, MBWE was also effective in increasing life satisfaction and reducing psychological distress among participants. Though participants revealed that after the course was over, they struggled with sustaining independent mindfulness practice, they noted that they had made specific health behavior changes because of it, such as increased physical activity.

Mindful Apps Specifically for Teachers

Though many of the mindfulness apps overviewed in both Chapter 3 and the parent section of this chapter can be useful for teachers for personal use, the following are apps that have greater applicability for educators in the classroom. Table 8.2 is not considered exhaustive, and technology is ever changing, so this list should be considered simply an introduction to some of the resources available to teachers.

Table 8.2 Mindfulness apps for teachers.

Name	Description
Calm.com (2022)	Calm is designed to help reduce stress and anxiety and promote better sleep through guided meditations, soothing music, and bedtime stories. Educators can access premium services for free through the Calm classroom initiative.
Mindful Scholar (Demo Mindful, 2022)	Provides suggested mindfulness techniques based on child's specific needs in the classroom. Flashcards, affirmations, and activities are also included.

Name	Description
ACT Companion: The Happiness Trap App (Berrick Psychology, 2022)	Assists users in engaging in positive action aligned with ACT through mindfulness exercises.
Headspace and Headspace for Educators (2022)	Includes guided mindfulness meditations and practices for adolescents and adults. Assists educators in engaging in mindfulness and incorporating mindfulness in their classrooms. Headspace for Educators provides free access to K–12 educators in the U.S., U.K., Canada, and Australia.
Smiling Mind (2022)	Provides a free mindfulness program for teachers focusing on stress, attention, well-being, and sleep among other topic areas.
Stop, Breathe & Think (2022)	Provides customized meditations based on how an individual is feeling at the moment. Separate programs are provided for children and adults. Educators receive free lifetime membership access.

ACT for Teachers and Other School Professionals

In addition to mindfulness intervention, ACT has been shown to be helpful for teachers in reducing stress and improving wellness and self-efficacy. A key finding across studies is that ACT increases teachers' psychological flexibility, which can aid in decreased experiential avoidance, higher levels of acceptance of circumstances, and increased effectiveness in their jobs (Biglan et al., 2013). Have a mental health professional run an in-service training or workshop on ACT digestible for school personnel as one way to begin exposing the material to staff. Content could include the six components of ACT and their applicability for both professional and personal use. The importance of psychological flexibility, the use of mindfulness, and values-based goal setting can all be incorporated into such a training. Engaging staff in experiential exercises aimed at demonstrating each of these components is recommended, as this is a particularly effective way to introduce the various ACT principles. Examples of easy to digest exercises include the Clipboard Technique, the Milk exercise, the Chinese Finger Trap, Leaves on a Stream meditation, and the 80th Birthday Party. All of these activities are overviewed in Chapter 4.

ACT Bibliotherapy. Teachers and staff can be encouraged to read a book about ACT for personal use as a way of enhancing psychological well-being. In a study by Jeffcoat and Hayes (2012), ACT bibliotherapy was used as an intervention with K–12 school personnel. Pre-intervention, three-fourths of the participants were above clinical cutoffs in impaired general mental health, depression, anxiety, or stress. Participants who read *Get Out of Your Mind & Into Your Life* (Hayes & Smith, 2005) for two months, including completing the exercises and quizzes, showed significant improvement in psychological health, including reduced stress, anxiety, and depressive symptoms, as compared to the wait-list control group. These findings lend support to the utility of self-study as an intervention. Given this, schools could consider having a brief in-service on the topic of ACT, then provide a workbook, such as *ACT Made Simple* by Harris (2009), *Burnout and Trauma Related Employment Stress: Acceptance and Commitment Strategies in the Helping Professions* by Holland et al. (2021), or *Get Out of Your Mind and Into Your Life* by Hayes and Smith (2005), for individual practice at home. Weekly or monthly meetings could be scheduled where the content and activities are discussed as they apply to the teachers' experiences.

Mindfulness and ACT for Educator Burnout and Compassion Fatigue

Teachers' psychological health is important for both their personal well-being and also for their capacity to effectively mentor and teach students. Because their work puts them in situations that are often stressful and challenging, they are more at risk for burnout. Burnout is a cumulative process marked by emotional exhaustion and withdrawal. It is associated with increased workload and institutional stress. Common symptoms of burnout include a reduced sense of personal accomplishment or meaning in work, mental exhaustion, isolation, depersonalization, and physical exhaustion (American Institute of Stress, 2018). Additionally, at times, teachers are in situations where they see or hear about the ongoing suffering of their students. Teachers working in schools with fewer resources and higher rates of community or family violence and poverty can find themselves overextended and overwhelmed by the needs of their students. In these circumstances, teachers may begin to experience extreme states of tension. They may be preoccupied with the suffering of their students, to the degree that it creates a type of secondary traumatic stress, also known as compassion fatigue (Figley, 1995). Compassion fatigue can be comorbid with burnout and be caused by exposure to one stressful/traumatic situation or be due to cumulative exposure to stressors/trauma. Compassion fatigue symptoms can include nervous system arousal, including trouble sleeping; isolation and loss of morale; decreased cognitive ability and judgment; loss of meaning, hope, and self-worth; problems with emotional modulation; fears around safety; trust and control issues; and problems with anger, depression, and anxiety. Additionally, the potential risk for acquiring symptoms of post-traumatic stress disorder (PTSD) symptoms is elevated (American Institute of Stress, 2018). Prevention of burnout and compassion fatigue, along with early intervention methods, are crucial to maintaining the mental well-being of educators and healthy classroom environments.

Creating a positive classroom environment is one avenue for preventing burnout. It includes increasing educator mindfulness practices, fostering supportive relationships with students, and focusing on positivity and gratitude in the classroom (Jennings, 2015). Mindfulness exercises including deep breathing, mindful activity, and heartfulness, (overviewed in Chapters 4 and 7) can be practiced in the classroom and woven throughout the school day. Focusing on techniques for mindful listening and compassion in the classroom can help both teacher and students build a supportive community of learners (Jennings, 2015). Additionally, gratitude has been found to be a buffer against burnout. Chan (2011) investigated an intervention focused on fostering gratitude amongst teachers and its effect on burnout. Results found that participants in the intervention had increased positive affect and satisfaction with their jobs and life, especially among those who were lower on dispositional gratitude. Various ways to increase gratitude, and heartfulness are discussed previously and in Chapter 3. Individuals who are grateful tend to be more helpful, forgiving, empathetic, and supportive toward others (McCullough et al., 2002), key traits in successful mentoring of others.

ACT is also helpful for reducing educator burnout. Experiential avoidance, the tendency to avoid painful or challenging internal experiences, is a common symptom of burnout. It's important to acknowledge and address challenges and issues, as opposed to avoiding or ignoring them. A focus of ACT work is to move participants toward psychological flexibility and acceptance of circumstances in order to set healthy, value-centered goals. ACT has been found to increase psychological flexibility and decrease experiential avoidance, stress, and burnout in teachers (Hinds et al., 2015). This idea has been validated through other research studies (Brinkborg et al., 2011; Lloyd et al., 2013).

ACT metaphors and interventions, such as the clipboard technique overviewed in Chapter 4, can help reduce experiential avoidance and cognitive fusion (key ingredients in burnout). Increasing mindful awareness of the situation, including the educator's own emotional experience, can assist in reducing reactivity and stress. Additionally, it's helpful to focus on the values that brought teachers into the profession. From this point, it's possible to set attainable short-term goals based on their values (a key component in ACT) and so reduce professional burnout.

A common ACT acceptance activity, described for children in Chapter 4, can also be used with adults. It's called the Flip Side of the Paper, also known as Two Sides of the Coin (Hayes & Greco, 2008). An adaptation of this exercise for teachers is provided here:

PRACTITIONER: (provide the teacher with a piece of blank paper). *With this piece of paper, I want you on one side to write down the thing about your job that you are struggling with the most. For example, I know you mentioned you have been having a hard time with not being given enough resources in order to do the projects you would like to do in the classroom. So, if this is what you choose, write down on one side of your paper, "not enough resources." If it is around disruptive behaviors in your classroom, you would write down "disruptive behaviors."*

TEACHER: *OK.* (teacher writes a struggle down on their paper)

PRACTITIONER: *Good. Ok, now flip your paper over. On this other side of the paper, I want you to write down the life area that you value that relates to this challenge. For example, you would likely write, "my career" or "teaching at this school" down as your life area.*

TEACHER: (writes down life area on the other side).

PRACTITIONER: *OK, now if I gave you the power to do so, would you crumple up and throw away the paper? You would be getting rid of the problem, but along with it you would also be giving up the other side too, as they are linked.*

TEACHER: *No! I love my job here at this school. I don't want to leave.*

PRACTITIONER: *OK, well, that is information for you. Sometimes when I do this exercise with people, they do want to crumple up the paper. That means the thing they are doing may no longer be in alignment with their values and so a change is necessary. However, you want to continue at your job. So, instead, let's do some work around how much attachment there is for you right now around this problem area. We can focus on some exercises to help move you to a place of acceptance around the issue.*

At this point the practitioner will want to introduce more activities and metaphors, such as Passengers on the Bus (Chapter 5), in order to help the educator continue to move in the direction of their valued goal, while reducing their attachment to the negative challenges along the way.

Mindfulness With Parents and Other Caregivers

Mindfulness has been used when working with parents and other caregivers to assist their own mental well-being, stress levels, and parenting abilities. Just as with children, mindfulness practices have been successfully used to intervene in stress reactions, mood disorders, inattention, and anxiety in adult populations (Khoury et al., 2015). It has long been understood that parent mental wellness is related to their children's functioning and sense of well-being (Piehler et al., 2014). Therefore, strengthening the mental health of parents through mindfulness techniques can positively impact the health of their families. Mindfulness practices have been found to have wide applicability. They have the potential to alleviate some of the stress of parenting preschoolers (Bluth & Wahler, 2011), to reduce parental over-reactivity and the strain of raising older children, and to cope with the challenges of parenting youth with attention deficit hyperactivity disorder and oppositional defiant disorder (Modesto-Lowe et al., 2014; van der Oord et al., 2012).

Mindfulness can not only be used to improve individual parent well-being, but can also be integrated into more traditional behavioral parent training (e.g., using strategic attention, applying reinforcements; Holland et al., 2017). A study conducted by Coatsworth et al. (2015) provides intriguing evidence for the unique contribution of mindfulness to standard parent training, with mindfulness activities boosting and better sustaining the effects of standard intervention. In a confirmatory factor analysis of an assessment measure for mindfulness in parenting (the Interpersonal Mindfulness in Parenting Scale (IMPS); Duncan, 2007), four factors were found to load into the construct of mindful parenting: present-centered attention, present-centered emotional awareness, non-judgmental acceptance, and non-reactivity (Duncan, 2007). These factors make intuitive sense; healthy parenting, being present and having emotional awareness, acceptance, and non-reactivity are all important skills for parents. This has been subsequently supported in the literature. In research conducted by Parent, McKee, Anton, et al. (2016), the IMPS was used to further investigate the effects of mindfulness in parenting and co-parenting relationships with a sample of 485 parents. Results found dispositional parental mindfulness was indirectly related to higher levels of positive parenting practices and lower levels of negative parenting practices. The authors noted that parent attunement and attention to the present moment in aspects of daily life impacted their parenting through their compassion, increased awareness, and reduced reactivity toward their children.

The idea of dispositional mindfulness in parenting not only has been shown to impact the parent-child relationship but was also found to be a mediating factor in internalizing and externalizing disorders for children. A study of 615 parents of youth across three developmental stages (young childhood, middle childhood, and adolescence) found higher levels of parent dispositional mindfulness were indirectly related to lower levels of youth internalizing and externalizing problems. This was consistent across all three life stages. These results suggest higher levels of mindful parenting are related to lower levels of negative parenting practices, which can in turn impact the individual well-being of a child. The replication of these findings across families with children at different developmental stages in this study lends support to the generalizability of these results (Parent, McKee, Rough, et al., 2016). The disposition of being mindful can be cultivated through practice and repetition, with the individual learning flexible new ways of approaching thoughts, feelings, and situations (Ritchhart & Perkins, 2000).

Many parents find mindfulness to be a relatively simple concept to understand but have difficulties when trying to use it in their daily interactions with their child. Remind parents that mindfulness is a skill that requires cultivation through regular practice, and it takes time to use it more fluidly. Psychoeducation can be an important initial step in introducing mindfulness to parents. Discuss with parents the impact of parental stress and from where the stress comes; this can be a validating conversation. The evolution of parenting, including the fact that the nuclear family is an aberration in the history of human beings, can be enlightening for parents. Pre-1950s children were raised in communities that included many stakeholders, with multiple trusted and highly motivated caretakers being involved in the child's care. In the post-World War II era, many families became isolated, with one parent (typically the mother) staying home and raising the children independently, with the other going to work. We are not adapted to be sole caregivers of children. Parental anxiety, in part, is due to this deviation from our ancestors (e.g., we were not meant to do it alone; Bögels & Restifo, 2014). Additionally, as students are pushed to be "super students" (pressured to achieve academically and extracurricularly; Kohn, 2006) parents have also been driven to be "super parents." They often feel compelled to be overly involved in their children's lives, arranging everything from playdates to extracurricular programs to fill their child's time with stimulation and further child resume building. These phenomena appear to be most prevalent in the United States among the middle class and the upper middle class; they are less common in other industrialized countries, such as Sweden and Germany (Doepke & Zilibotti, 2019). Helping parents understand this gives them more choice in how they parent and helps loosen the grip of the guilt parents inevitably experience for not being "perfect." Psychoeducation with parents can also include what happens biologically and neurologically in the body and brain when under stress, and how mindfulness can help to decrease this activation of the sympathetic nervous system (see Chapter 3 for more information).

Exercises that can be integrated into a parent's daily life, such as mindful breathing, mindful eating, and mindful walking, are relatively easy to practice and more tangible initially than some meditative techniques. Identifying regular activities in which parents are already engaging can increase the likelihood they will practice mindfulness skills more often (Holland et al., 2017). These skills are all overviewed in Chapter 3 and can be used with adults.

Breathwork is an example of a structured exercise that can be introduced to parents as a way to practice mindfulness (Bögels & Restifo, 2014). The 4x8 breathing technique overviewed in Chapter 3 can be easily adapted for use with parents. To begin, instruct parents to get into a comfortable seated position and have them either soften their gaze or close their eyes. Model for them taking in deep breaths in to the count of four through their nose, and out to the count of eight through their mouth. As they practice this skill, encourage them to focus their attention on their breath, noticing any bodily sensations that may be occurring throughout (e.g., the temperature of the air as it enters/exits their nose, the rise and fall of their chest/stomach, etc.). During this time, the idea of thought bubbles could be introduced. If parents notice thoughts, as they likely will, they should acknowledge these thoughts, then allow those thoughts to float away, gently bringing their attention back to their breath. An added exercise could be the use of the 5 Senses Script, as outlined in Chapter 3.

Encourage parents to find groups and self-study materials to continue mindfulness practices on their own. Recommending books such as *Buddha's Brain* by Hanson and Mendius (2009) and *Mindful Parenting* by Race (2014), or the mindfulness apps covered throughout this chapter (e.g., Head Space or Calm) can be useful for parents who would like outside readings and support.

Parent Work and ACT

Practitioners can promote ACT principles when working with parents through the use of metaphors and specific exercises. In a case example by Coyne and Wilson (2004), ACT was successfully integrated with parent-child interactional therapy (PCIT) with the mother of a typically developing six-year-old child exhibiting conduct problems (e.g., aggression and noncompliance). The mother was experiencing a great deal of embarrassment and anxiety around her son's behavior, impeding her ability to parent effectively. The mother was initially provided with several training sessions focused on ACT principles, including mindfulness, values identification, cognitive defusion, and acceptance prior to participating in PCIT coaching sessions focused on parenting skills. Values identification was used to increase treatment engagement and committed action exercises were incorporated to facilitate participation in the PCIT coaching sessions. Other ACT principles, such as cognitive defusion, were woven throughout the PCIT training. For example, the child's mother had difficulties adhering to some behavioral principles due to thoughts about her incompetence and fears about her child's future. At the end of the training, not only was her child exhibiting lower aggression levels and less noncompliant behavior, but the mother reported a significant decrease in her own level of anxiety and an increased sense of confidence and effectiveness in parenting.

The following section offers practical suggestions on how to incorporate several key ACT principles into working with parents. As overviewed in previous chapters, ACT includes six core components: Contact with the Present Moment (Mindfulness), Cognitive Defusion, Acceptance, Self-as-Context, Values, and Committed Action. Each of these will be discussed as it relates to working with parents.

Contact With the Present Moment (Mindfulness)

Experiential avoidance is a tendency to attempt to avoid or suppress unwanted experiences, feelings, or thoughts. When parenting, experiential avoidance can lead to inflexible parenting strategies, overreacting to the child's behavior, being inconsistent with consequences, and ultimately withdrawing from the child (Coyne & Murrell, 2009). Mindfulness-based parenting encourages parents to be present, nonreactive, and to have awareness of circumstances, as opposed to being experientially avoidant of them. It aims to cultivate empathy, patience, and persistence in the face of adversity (Race, 2014). The mindfulness techniques used with parents mentioned earlier in this chapter are all relevant to this component of ACT.

Cognitive Defusion

It is common for people to focus their attention on the contents of their mind (thoughts, memories, assumptions, beliefs, images, etc.) rather than what is experienced through the five senses. Decisions and actions are, therefore, often based on one's internal experience (thoughts, memories, etc.) rather than what is actually going on around them. These internal experiences can become rigid. They are often a primary lens through which situations are experienced. Harris (2009) notes that in this state of cognitive fusion, thoughts can seem like absolute truth or rules one must follow. In parenting, these rules and labels can impact the parent's ability to cope and function. Take, for example, the following passage offered by Coyne and Wilson (2004, p. 470).

An Adapted Zen Koan for Parents

Question 1. What is the sound of one hand clapping?
Answer: The sound of one hand clapping is the sound of one hand clapping.
Question 2: What is the sound of one child misbehaving?
Answer: The sound of one child misbehaving is the sound of one child misbehaving.
Question 3: What is the sound of my child misbehaving?
Answer: The sound of "I cannot control my child," the sound of "I should be able to," the sound of "I am a bad parent," the sound of "I don't know what to do," the sound of "I hate this child," the sound of "I should not feel this way," and the sound of my failure.

This passage powerfully illustrates how cognitive fusion can negatively impact parenting perception and behaviors. Note the "I am" labels and the clouding of experience by negative thoughts. Those thoughts will likely interfere with subsequent parenting decisions. In ACT, the content of the thought is not what is problematic; instead, it is the parent's relationship or "fusion" with the thought that is a problem. For example, a parent has the thought "I cannot control my child," and, as a result, struggles to initiate effective discipline practices due to perceived ineffectiveness. The parent would be considered cognitively fused with the thought. In contrast, a parent has the same thought and acknowledges it as just a thought, and nothing more. They would be less cognitively fused and more likely to use effective discipline tactics with their child (Holland et al., 2017).

Cognitive fusion, as described in earlier chapters, is intricately related to words that people tell themselves. This can interfere with the ability to clearly see situations or circumstances. For instance, we might think of the word "worthless" and then think about our inability to perform a function at our job. By extension we then begin to associate the word "worthless" with other areas of our life, such as parenting, or to our life as a whole. A commonly used defusion technique that could be introduced to parents is the "Milk" technique (Tichener, 1916); parents would quickly repeat the word "milk" over and over again for a minute in rapid succession. This action, over time, weakens the attachment between the word and its meaning. The literal meaning of the word dissipates until the word becomes simply noise. This technique can then be used on words that may be triggering, such as "worthless" or "failure" to loosen those associations.

Acceptance

When individuals try to push away their pain, also known as experiential avoidance, they add stress to their experience. Instead of just experiencing the pain of the situation, they now experience pain and stress, which heightens the discomfort (Bögels & Restifo, 2014). This holds true when a parent attempts to avoid or suppress unwanted thoughts, sensations and/or feelings about their child. This can result in use of ineffective parenting strategies (e.g., withdrawal, punitive/controlling style, inconsistent parenting, etc.). Acceptance is an alternative to experiential avoidance (Hayes et al., 2012). By supporting parents to become more accepting of their experiences, they will be better able to mindfully parent (Holland et al., 2017).

When introducing acceptance, it is helpful to first acknowledge the futility of avoidance (Holland et al., 2017). Tolle (1999) notes that which we resist, persists. When we avoid issues or challenges, they tend to become more pronounced or lead to other problems. Highlight that acceptance is not the same thing as agreeing with or consenting. Instead, it is no longer avoiding and having a willingness to acknowledge a challenging thought, feeling, or situation. Only then are we able to choose what to do next. Without this acknowledgment, we become stuck in experiential avoidance (McCurry, 2009). Various metaphors have been developed in ACT to assist with this process (Hayes et al., 2012). Simple examples that highlight the futility of the struggle (e.g., experiential avoidance) include getting caught in quicksand, playing tug-of-war, or having fingers stuck in a Chinese finger trap. In each of these situations, the more a parent struggles, the worse it becomes (Holland et al., 2017).

After parents recognize the ineffectiveness of experiential avoidance, the practitioner can introduce the idea of acceptance as an alternative. Letting go of the struggle with negative thoughts and feelings gives parents energy to focus on more effective parenting strategies. The Passengers on the Bus metaphor (Hayes et al., 2012), adapted for parents, can be helpful here. Encourage parents to think of themselves as the bus driver, and the passengers as their troubling thoughts, feelings, and memories. Parents want to drive their bus (their lives) toward a value-based goal (e.g., being a "good parent"). But there are times when the passengers become angry and challenge the bus driver, say hurtful comments, or demand that the bus be taken in a different direction. The bus driver may find themselves arguing with the passengers and feel overwhelmed, distracted, or flooded by their presence. Alternatively, they may strike a deal that they will drive the bus wherever the passengers want, so long as they sit back and stay quiet, or they may try and push the passengers off the bus. Discuss the experience of being overwhelmed by thoughts, feelings, and experiences about parenting, along with the process of experiential avoidance. The challenge is for parents to consider the benefits of simply acknowledging and accepting the passengers on their bus while they remain at the controls. They can continue to drive the bus in the direction the parent themselves would like to go.

Self-as-Context

In ACT, self-as-context means that we are not the content of our experiences; we are not our thoughts, our feelings, the images that pass through our minds, or our experienced sensations. Through activities and metaphors designed to decrease cognitive fusion, and increase mindfulness and acceptance, we can see ourselves as an observing self, as opposed to defining ourselves as the content of the stories we tell ourselves (Hayes et al., 2012).

The following is an adapted activity that can be practiced by parents in order to help with the idea of self-as-context as offered by Tolle (1999):

> *Stop and quietly listen to what you are saying to yourself, to the voice in your head. Now ask yourself the following two questions:*
>   *Am I the thoughts that are going through my head?*
>   *Or, am I the one who is aware of these thoughts that are going through my head?*

This exercise helps parents distinguish themselves from their thoughts, becoming less fused with their cognitions and "I am" statements. These "I am" statements are known as self-as-content in ACT

(Hayes et al., 2012). When parents are suffering, they often have a sense of themselves based upon their past experiences or future fears, (e.g., "I am a bad parent," or "I will be a failure in parenting."). Once parents are less entangled with their thoughts, they can begin to recognize that they are not their thoughts and emotions; rather, there is a *stable self* that observes. From this perspective, parents can learn to let go of unhelpful self-evaluations, while retaining their sense of themselves (Holland et al., 2017). This process in ACT is known as self-as-context, which is a form of perspective taking (Hayes et al., 2012).

Values

Values are our principles, the ideals that give our lives direction and meaning. These principles and ideals tell us where to direct our energies in work, recreation, and relationships (e.g., goal formation; McCurry, 2009). For example, parents may wish to "be a good parent." This value would then direct their behaviors (e.g., helping their child with their homework, making breakfast for their child, volunteering at their child's extracurricular event, etc.). Remembering their values can assist parents in making decisions that they may find challenging or aversive. For example, parents may find it easier to implement a timeout procedure, which can be time-intensive and emotionally aversive, by reminding themselves of their parenting values (e.g., raising a well-behaved child; Holland et al., 2017).

There are various ways parents can clarify their values. Use a values list or rank values, as offered in Hayes and Smith (2005). Some of the most common value areas for adults are:

marriage, couple, or other intimate relationship;
parenting;
family relations;
friendship and social relations;
career and employment;
education. training, personal growth, and development;
recreation and leisure;
spirituality;
citizenship; and
health and physical well-being.

As parents assess how these areas rank in importance in their lives in the moment, they can then begin to construct goals that are meaningful to them. A technique for identifying values is the 80th Birthday Party (Hayes & Smith, 2005), as described in Chapter 4. Parents are asked to imagine themselves at their 80th birthday party, and then asked to imagine what their children would stand up to say about them in a speech. Be sure to have the speech contain what the parent stood for and valued in their parenting role. These speeches usually align with what the parent values.

Committed Action

Committed action means purposefully engaging in values-based activities, even those that are difficult. Over time, a pattern of action is deliberately created that serves the value (Hayes et al., 2012). For instance, if the parent values raising a child who is independent, then the parent would deliberately choose to have their child try some things on their own before stepping in to help (e.g., picking up their room). Parents should be aware of barriers to implementing their goal, such as their child whining or having a tantrum. A commitment to action also means refraining from experiential avoidance (e.g., picking up the room for their child, giving up, etc.) and using mindfulness and cognitive defusion techniques to help with the discomfort involved in their child's behavior (Holland et al., 2017).

Case Examples

Jenni, Third-Grade Teacher

Jenni (she/her/hers), a third-grade teacher, came to her colleague Mr. Crane, the school psychologist, because she was experiencing increased fatigue and challenges concentrating. Mr. Crane had just given a presentation on burnout for educators at the Monday afternoon teacher's meeting, and Jenni recognized that many of her symptoms fell into the category of burnout. Upon hearing Jenni's concerns, Mr. Crane offered to help Jenni get started on some wellness practices and to connect her to resources. He encouraged Jenni to call their employee assistance program (EAP) to gain some increased support during this time since Jenni also mentioned she was beginning to feel depressed.

Mr. Crane practiced several mindfulness strategies with Jenni, such as 4x8 breathing and the 5 Senses Activity in order to interrupt her negative and repetitive thinking patterns. He encouraged her to begin reading the book, *Buddha's Brain* by Hanson and Mendius (2009) to assist with outside mindfulness exploration. Additionally, he encouraged Jenni to begin journaling a few nights per week before bed, writing down one thing she was grateful for that day, then reading her positive note to herself the next morning. She also downloaded the app "Headspace" on her smartphone and began a regular mindfulness practice using the app.

Jenni was also beginning to feel overwhelmed with some of her students' classroom behaviors, causing her to miss work at times because of how reactive she felt toward the situation. For this, Mr. Crane worked with Jenni on some acceptance strategies. He used the clipboard technique (Chapter 4) to decrease her cognitive fusion and increase her acceptance of her situation. He used the Flip Side of the Paper activity, to remind her of the values that brought her into the profession and to increase her acceptance of some of the challenges in her work. Additionally, he encouraged Jenni to read, *Get Out of Your Mind and Into Your Life* by Hayes and Smith (2005), for individual practice at home.

Jenni followed up with Mr. Crane a month later, noting she felt significantly better, with more reported energy and increased concentration and positive mood. She had connected with a provider through her EAP program, who encouraged her to continue to use the mindfulness and acceptance practices suggested by Mr. Crane.

Felix, Father of Two Children

Felix (he/him/his), a father of two children, ages 9 and 14, approached his younger daughter's school counselor after an evening parent workshop on stress and parenting. Felix told the counselor that he felt hopeful in hearing the counselor speak about stress and how to best manage it as a parent. Felix had been feeling isolated as a single father of his two children and overwhelmed with responsibilities at work and home. He told the counselor that, at times, he felt like he was failing at both roles and had a lot of anxiety. Felix also said that his anxiety was beginning to affect his children; he was becoming more irritable and distant with them.

The school counselor first introduced Felix to some mindfulness exercises, such as 4x8 breathing and alternate nostril breathing (A.N.B.) to help reduce his physiological reactivity of stress and anxiety. He also encouraged him to use the Calm app to support Felix's breathwork at home. Felix agreed to work on these mindfulness activities, sharing them with his children to support a family practice of the techniques. Felix and the counselor decided to meet again the next week to follow up.

Upon return, Felix told the counselor that he did feel less stressed and calmer using the mindfulness techniques. However, his thoughts of being a "failure" were still quite frequent. The counselor introduced Felix to ACT, specifically the idea of cognitive defusion. Together they discussed the distortion behind "I Am" statements and they began to create flexibility in his thinking via the Milk technique, and through the Leaves on a Stream meditation (Chapter 4). Through these techniques, Felix began to see that his thoughts were just thoughts, not facts, and he began to experience more control detaching from them. At this point, the school counselor helped Felix identify what he most values in his life. He named his family, his work, and his health. Together the counselor and Felix created short-term goals based on these valued areas.

Felix returned to give the school counselor an update a month later. Felix noted less stress and anxiety and more motivation at home and work. Felix said that he had also begun sharing the techniques he had learned with his children, and that together they began a nightly mindfulness practice at bedtime.

Conclusion

The mental health of parents, caregivers, and educators is integral to children's healthy development. The need to support parents and educators, within the context of providing mental health support to youth, is becoming well-supported by research. As evident from the research, mindfulness and ACT are two approaches that can assist in parent and teacher well-being.

References

Ackerman, C. (2017, December 5). *9 self-compassion exercises & worksheets for increasing compassion.* PositivePsychology.com. https://positivepsychology.com/self-compassion-exercises-worksheets/

American Institute of Stress. (2018). *Compassion fatigue.* www.stress.org/military/for-practitionersleaders/compassion-fatigue

Berrick Psychology. (2022). *ACT companion: The Happiness Trap App* (Version 3.8) [Mobile app]. Mac App Store. https://apps.apple.com/us/app/act-companion-happiness-trap/id668468577

Biglan, A., Layton, G. L., Jones, L. B., Hankins, M., & Rusby, J. C. (2013). The value of workshops on psychological flexibility for early childhood special education staff. *Topics in Early Childhood Special Education, 32*(4), 196–210.

Bluth, K., & Wahler, R. G. (2011). Parenting preschoolers: Can mindfulness help? *Mindfulness, 2*(4), 282–285.

Bögels, S., & Restifo, K. (2014). *Mindful parenting: A guide for mental health practitioners.* W. W. Norton & Co.

Brinkborg, H., Michanek, J., Hesser, H., & Berglund, G. (2011). Acceptance and commitment therapy for the treatment of stress among social workers: A randomized controlled trial. *Behaviour Research and Therapy, 49*(6–7), 389–398.

Brown School of Public Health. (2019). *Mindfulness Center at Brown.* www.brown.edu/public-health/mindfulness/node/1

Calm.com. (2022). *Calm.* (Version 5.37.1) [Mobile app]. Mac App Store. https://apps.apple.com/us/app/calm/id571800810

Chan, D. (2011). Burnout and life satisfaction: Does gratitude intervention make a difference among Chinese school teachers in Hong Kong? *Educational Psychology, 31*(7), 809–823.

Coatsworth, J. D., Duncan, L. G., Nix, R. L., Greenberg, M. T., Gayles, J. G., Bamberger, K. T., Berrena, E., & Demi, M. A. (2015). Integrating mindfulness with parent training: Effects of the mindfulness-enhanced strengthening families program. *Developmental Psychology, 51*(1), 26–35.

Coyne, L. W., & Murrell, A. R. (2009). *The joy of parenting: An acceptance and commitment therapy guide to effective parenting in the early years.* New Harbinger Publications.

Coyne, L. W., & Wilson, K. G. (2004). The role of cognitive fusion in impaired parenting: An RFT analysis. *International Journal of Psychology and Psychological Therapy, 4*(3), 469–486.

Demo Mindful. (2022). *Mindful scholar* (Version 1.1) [Mobile app]. Mac App Store. https://apps.apple.com/us/app/mindful-scholar/id1447526683

Doepke, M., & Zilibotti, F. (2019, February 22). The parent trap: The greater a country's income inequality, the likelier parents are to push their kids to work hard. *The Washington Post.* www.washingtonpost.com/news/postevery thing/wp/2019/02/22/feature/how-economic-inequality-gives-rise-to-hyper-paren ting/

Duncan, L. G. (2007). *Assessment of mindful parenting among parents of early adolescents: Development and validation of the interpersonal mindfulness in parenting scale* [Doctoral dissertation]. Penn State Electronic Theses and Dissertations for Graduate School. https://etda.libraries.psu.edu/files/final_submissions/ 3737

Emerson, L. M., Leyland, A., Hudson, K., Rowse, G., Hanley, P., & Hugh-Jones, S. (2017). Teaching mindfulness to teachers: A systematic review and narrative synthesis. *Mindfulness, 8*(5), 1136–1149.

Emmons, R. A., & McCullough, M. E. (2003). Counting blessings versus burdens: An experimental investigation of gratitude and subjective well-being in daily life. *Journal of Personality and Social Psychology, 84*(2), 377–389.

Figley, C. R. (Ed.). (1995). *Brunner/Mazel psychological stress series, No. 23. Compassion fatigue: Coping with secondary traumatic stress disorder in those who treat the traumatized.* Brunner/Mazel.

Garrison Institute. (2019, December 19). *Cultivating awareness and resilience in education (CARE) for teachers.* www.garrisoninstitute.org/what-were-working-on/ care-for-the-caregivers/care-for-teachers/

Hanson, R., & Mendius, R. (2009). *Buddha's brain: The practical neuroscience of happiness, love, and wisdom.* New Harbinger Publication.

Harris, A. R., Jennings, P. A., Katz, D. A., Abenavoli, R. M., & Greenberg, M. T. (2016). Promoting stress management and wellbeing in educators: Feasibility and efficacy of a school-based yoga and mindfulness intervention. *Mindfulness, 7*(1), 143–154.

Harris, R. (2009). *ACT made simple: A quick start guide to ACT basics and beyond.* New Harbinger Publication.

Hayes, S. C., & Greco, L. A. (2008). Acceptance and mindfulness for youth: It's time. In L. A. Greco & S. C. Hayes (Eds.), *Acceptance & mindfulness treatments for children and adolescents: A practitioner's guide* (pp. 3–13). New Harbinger Publication.

Hayes, S. C., & Smith, S. (2005). *Get out of your mind and into your life: The new acceptance and commitment therapy.* New Harbinger Publications.

Hayes, S. C., Strosahl, K. D., & Wilson, K. G. (2012). *Acceptance and commitment therapy: An experiential approach to behavior change* (2nd ed.). Guilford Press.

Headspace Inc. (2022). *Headspace* (Version 3.209.0) [Mobile app]. Mac app store. https://apps.apple.com/us/app/headspace-mindful-meditation/id4931 45008

Hinds, E., Jones, L. B., Gau, J. M., Forrester, K. K., & Biglan, A. (2015). Teacher distress and the role of experiential avoidance. *Psychology in the Schools, 52*(3), 284–297.

Holland, M. L., Brock, S. E., Oren, T., & van Eckhardt, M. (2021). *Burnout and trauma related employment stress: Acceptance and commitment strategies in the helping professions.* Springer.

Holland, M. L., Hawks, J., & Gimpel Peacock, G. (2017). *Emotional and behavioral problems of young children: Effective interventions in the preschool and kindergarten year* (2nd ed.). Guilford Press.

Jeffcoat, T., & Hayes, S. C. (2012). A randomized trial of ACT bibliotherapy on the mental health of K-12 teachers and staff. *Behaviour Research and Therapy, 50*(9), 571–579.

Jennings, P. A. (2015). *Mindfulness for teachers: Simple skills for peace and productivity in the classroom (the Norton series on the social neuroscience of education).* W.W. Norton & Company.

Jennings, P. A., Brown, J. L., Frank, J. L., Doyle, S., Oh, Y., Davis, R., Rasheed, D., DeWeese, A., DeMauro, A. A., Cham, H., & Greenberg, M. T. (2017). Impacts of the CARE for teachers program on teachers' social and emotional competence and classroom interactions. *Journal of Educational Psychology, 109*(7), 1010–1028.

Khoury, B., Sharma, M., Rush, S. E., & Fournier, C. (2015). Mindfulness-based stress reduction for healthy individuals: A meta-analysis. *Journal of Psychosomatic Research, 78*(6), 519–528.

Klimecki, O. M., Leiberg, S., Lamm, C., & Singer, T. (2013). Functional neural plasticity and associated changes in positive affect after compassion training. *Cerebral Cortex, 23*(7), 1552–1561.

Kohn, A. (2006). *The homework myth: Why our kids get too much of a bad thing.* Da Capo Press.

Lloyd, J., Bond, F. W., & Flaxman, P. E. (2013). The value of psychological flexibility: Examining psychological mechanisms underpinning a cognitive behavioural therapy intervention for burnout. *Work & Stress, 27*(2), 181–199.

McCullough, M. E., Emmons, R. A., & Tsang, J. A. (2002). The grateful disposition: A conceptual and empirical topography. *Journal of Personality and Social Psychology, 82*(1), 112–127.

McCurry, C. (2009). *Parenting your anxious child with mindfulness and acceptance: A powerful new approach to overcoming fear, panic, and worry using acceptance and commitment therapy.* New Harbinger Publications.

Modesto-Lowe, V., Chaplin, M., Godsay, V., & Soovajian, V. (2014). Parenting teens with attention-deficit/hyperactivity disorder: Challenges and opportunities. *Clinical Pediatrics, 53*(10), 943–948.

Nosaka, M., & Okamura, H. (2015). A single session of an integrated yoga program as a stress management tool for school employees: Comparison of daily practice and nondaily practice of a yoga therapy program. *The Journal of Alternative and Complementary Medicine, 21*(7), 444–449.

Parent, J., McKee, L. G., Anton, M., Gonzalez, M., Jones, D. J., & Forehand, R. (2016). Mindfulness in parenting and coparenting. *Mindfulness, 7*(2), 504–513.

Parent, J., McKee, L. G., Rough, J. N., & Forehand, R. (2016). The association of parent mindfulness with parenting and youth psychopathology across three developmental stages. *Journal of Abnormal Child Psychology, 44*(1), 191–202.

Passage Works. (2014). *Stress management and relaxation techniques in education (SMART)*. http://passageworks.org/courses/smart-in-education/

Piehler, T. F., Lee, S. S., Bloomquist, M. L., & August, G. J. (2014). Moderating effects of parental well-being on parenting efficacy outcomes by intervention delivery model of the early risers conduct problems prevention program. *The Journal of Primary Prevention, 35*(5), 321–337.

Poulin, P. A. (2009). *Mindfulness-based wellness education: A longitudinal evaluation with students in initial teacher education* [Doctoral dissertation, University of Toronto]. University of Toronto TSpace. https://tspace.library.utoronto.ca/handle/1807/26538

Race, K. (2014). *Mindful parenting: Simple and powerful solutions for raising creative, engaged, happy kids in today's hectic world.* St. Martin's Griffin.

Ritchhart, R., & Perkins, D. N. (2000). Life in the mindful classroom: Nurturing the disposition of mindfulness. *Journal of Social Issues, 56*(1), 27–47.

Roeser, R. W., Schonert-Reichl, K. A., Jha, A., Cullen, M., Wallace, L., Wilensky, R., Oberle, E., Thomson, K., Taylor, C., & Harrison, J. (2013). Mindfulness training and reductions in teacher stress and burnout: Results from two randomized, waitlist-control field trials. *Journal of Educational Psychology, 105*(3), 787–804.

Smiling Mind. (2022). *Smiling mind: Meditation for all ages* (Version 4.10.0) [Mobile app]. Mac App Store. https://apps.apple.com/us/app/smiling-mind/id560442518

Stop, Breathe & Think. (2022). *Stop breathe think: Meditation* (Version 10.3) [Mobile app]. Mac App Store. https://apps.apple.com/us/app/stop-breathe-think-meditation/id778848692

Taylor, C., Harrison, J., Haimovitz, K., Oberle, E., Thomson, K., Schonert-Reichl, K., & Roeser, R. W. (2016). Examining ways that a mindfulness-based intervention reduces stress in public school teachers: A mixed-methods study. *Mindfulness, 7*(6), 1449.

Tichener, E. B. (1916). *A text-book of psychology.* Macmillan.

Tolle, E. (1999). *The power of now: A guide to spiritual enlightenment.* New World Library.

van der Oord, S., Bögels, S. M., & Peijnenburg, D. (2012). The effectiveness of mindfulness training for children with ADHD and mindful parenting for their parents. *Journal of Child and Family Studies, 21*(1), 139–147.

9 Evaluating Outcomes and Conclusion

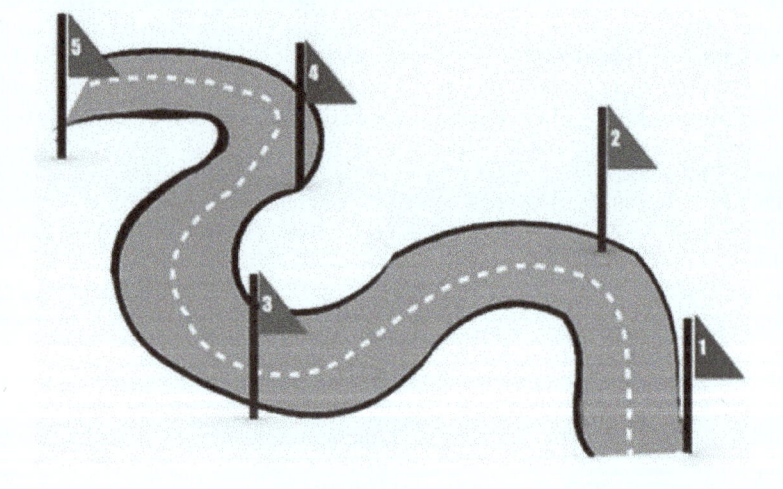

Roadmap to Chapter 9:
This chapter overviews how to evaluate the outcomes of your intervention. Specifically, it reviews:

- measures to assess for mindfulness in youth
- measures to assess for mindfulness in adults, and
- conclusions and future directions.

A critical aspect of intervention and program implementation is monitoring effectiveness. If time, energy, and resources are to be invested in an intervention, it is important to determine if the intervention is effective at reaching the goals that have been set. Additionally, not every population will respond to the intervention equally, and some adaptations or modifications may be necessary if the data reveals limited progress.

DOI: 10.4324/9781003318101-9

Measures to evaluate various aspects of mindfulness with youth have been developed. Ideally these assessments would be administered before, during, and after the intervention in order to determine effectiveness and assess progress. When choosing a measure, consider the type of intervention you are using (e.g., mindful breathing, acceptance techniques, etc.) and identify a measure that specifically targets this type of intervention. As noted in Chapter 2, mindfulness questionnaires do not always correlate with the intervention used (Manuel et al., 2017), and the underlying latent variable influencing the item responses on certain scales may be reflective of some variable other than mindfulness, such as inattentiveness or anxiety (Van Dam et al., 2010). To assist with this challenge, we recommend you assess for changes in mindfulness that are consistent with the intervention being used (e.g., meditation vs. yoga vs. ACT), as well as measure other areas with relevant assessments, (e.g., inattention, anxiety, depression). For example, if implementing an intervention classroom-wide or school-wide, consider assessing variables such as school attendance, disciplinary referrals, grades, and so on. This can help determine the wider impact of the intervention.

Specific mindfulness measures that can be used with youth and adults are overviewed next.

Mindfulness Rating Scales for Children and Adolescents

Typically, mindfulness research in the childhood population has relied on assessing target behaviors, as observed by key adult figures in a child's life. Outcome data have primarily focused on changes observed in problem behaviors (e.g., acting out, withdrawal, avoidance, inattention), as opposed to measuring the child's level of mindfulness and mindful practice. However, over the last several decades there has been an increase in the development of self-report mindfulness assessments for youth. Three of the more commonly used measures that are relevant for assessing mindfulness in youth are the Child Acceptance and Mindfulness Measure (CAMM; Greco et al., 2011), the Mindful Attention Awareness Scale-Adolescent (MAAS-A; Brown & Ryan, 2003), and the Mindful Thinking and Action Scale for Adolescents (MTSA; West et al., 2007). These are summarized in Table 9.1. Unfortunately, to date, there is not a well-validated measure for assessing mindfulness in children under age 10.

The CAMM (Greco et al., 2011) is a 10-item self-report measure designed to assess mindfulness on a 5-point scale (0 = *never true*, 4 = *always true*) for youth ages 10–17. Through factor analyses, a single-factor solution was chosen that covers present-moment awareness, as well as judgmental and nonaccepting responses to thoughts and feelings (Greco et al., 2011). Results from other studies confirm the one-dimensional factor structure of the American version of the CAMM and the internal

Table 9.1 Summary of youth mindfulness assessments.

Measure	Brief Description	Number of Items	Age Range
CAMM	A self-report assessment that measures present-moment awareness, as well as judgmental and nonaccepting responses to thoughts and feelings.	10	10–17 years old
MAAS-A	A self-report measure of trait mindfulness, with "presence" being emphasized as a key component.	14	14–18 years old
MTSA	A self-report measure of mindfulness across four subscales: healthy self-regulation (HSR), active attention, awareness-observation, and accepting experience.	32	13–17 years old

consistency (α= .84) of the ten CAMM items (Kuby et al., 2015; Sünbül, 2018). Good convergent and incremental validity has also been found when using the CAMM (Greco et al., 2011; Kuby et al., 2015). The CAMM has been validated in a variety of countries and in different languages. Of note is that research examining the use of the CAMM in some other countries found that the single-factor model is not well-supported and, instead, multifactorial models are a better fit. For example, the Italian version of the CAMM shows a two-factor solution, named "Awareness" and "Willingness" (Ristallo et al., 2016), whereas The Turkish version of the CAMM (Sünbül, 2018) and the Spanish version of the CAMM support the single factor model. The Spanish version, however, eliminated 5 of the 10 items (2, 3, 5, 6, and 10) from the original version, as these items were not predictive of mindfulness in the sample (Guerra et al., 2019). Some studies showed the CAMM may not be sensitive to meditation and yoga practice in children or may even show contrary outcomes in adolescents with prior meditation or yoga experience (e.g., de Bruin et al., 2011; de Bruin et al., 2014). More research in this area is needed. Overall, results suggest that the CAMM may be a useful measure of mindfulness skills for school-aged children and adolescents.

The **MAAS-A** (Brown et al., 2011) is a 14-item self-report measure designed to assess mindfulness in adolescents, ages 14–18. Items are answered on a 6-point scale (1= almost always, 6 = almost never), with higher numbers indicative of higher trait mindfulness. Items were adapted from the adult version of the MAAS (Brown & Ryan, 2003), with "presence" being emphasized as a key component (Brown et al., 2011). The MAAS-A showed good internal reliability (α= .82 – .84) in a general community sample, as well as with a sample of adolescents with anxiety and mood disorders (α= .86; Brown et al., 2011). Exploratory and confirmatory factor analyses substantiate a unidimensional structure (Brown et al., 2011; de Bruin et al., 2011), with males scoring slightly higher than females (consistent with past results with adult populations; Brown & Ryan, 2003). Replicated studies evidence the MAAS-A to have high internal consistency (de Bruin et al., 2011). Of note is that increases in MAAS-A scores among mindfulness-based stress reduction participants were significantly related to beneficial changes on external measures of psychological well-being and adaptive functioning in randomized trials (Brown et al., 2011). Other studies confirm this finding, with higher levels of mindfulness, as measured on the MAAS-A, negatively correlated with self-reported stress and maladaptive cognitions, such as rumination and catastrophizing, while being positively correlated with happiness and healthy self-regulation (de Bruin et al., 2011).

The MTSA (West et al., 2007) is a 32-item self-report measure of mindfulness for use with adolescents ages 13–17. Items are rated on a 5-point Likert scale across four subscales: healthy self-regulation (HSR), active attention, awareness-observation, and accepting experience. The HSR subscale has been used in studies validating other youth mindfulness measures, showing positive correlations with both the CAMM and MAAS-A (Brown et al., 2011; de Bruin et al., 2011). The MTASA has shown good internal consistency (α= .85), with subscale alphas ranging from .47 to .84 (West, 2008). Thus far, the MTASA has only been validated in non-clinical samples and, therefore, more research is needed in order to best understand the validity and utility of this measure, particularly when working with a clinical sample.

Mindfulness Rating Scales for Adults

Compared to youth, there are more mindfulness scales geared toward adults. A comprehensive review of these measures is beyond the scope of this chapter; however, commonly used rating scales are summarized in Table 9.2. We encourage the reader to further investigate the information and the psychometric properties of each scale to determine the best choice for their needs. Note that some of the scales measure trait mindfulness, while others measure state mindfulness. Trait mindfulness can be considered more of an ongoing, stable indicator of how mindful the individual is. State mindfulness inventories measure more transient mindfulness, typically resulting from engaging in a recent mindfulness practice.

These scales can be useful in tracking your mindful awareness and progress during your own practice or in adults with whom you are working. We recommend you try a variety of the measures located in Table 9.2 to determine which fits best. Be sure to determine what specific concepts of mindfulness you are interested in assessing and match

Table 9.2 Summary of adult mindfulness and acceptance assessments.

Measure	Brief Description
Cognitive and Affective Scale of Mindfulness-Revised (CAMS-R) (Feldman et al., 2007)	The CAMS-R takes a multi-dimensional view of trait mindfulness as a broad construct that includes four components: Attention; Present-focus; Awareness; Acceptance.
Five Facet Mindfulness Questionnaire (Baer et al., 2006).	A trait mindfulness measure that examines the following five facets of mindfulness: Nonreactivity to inner experiences; Observing/noticing/attending to sensations/perceptions/thoughts/feelings; Acting with awareness/automatic pilot/concentration/nondistraction; Describing/labeling with words; Nonjudging of experience.
Mindful Attention Awareness Scale (or MAAS) (Brown & Ryan, 2003)	The MAAS is a trait mindfulness scale that involves two components of consciousness: awareness and attention, which are then combined to create an overall score of mindlessness or mindfulness.
Freiburg Mindfulness Inventory (Walach et al., 2006)	The FMI assesses mindfulness as a process of regulating one's attention with the aim of approaching experiences with an open and nonjudgmental awareness, as well as curiosity and openness to the experience.
Langer Mindfulness Scale (Pirson et al., 2012)	Mindfulness on the Langer, a trait scale, is seen as a construct with four defining characteristics: Novelty seeking; Engagement; Novelty producing; and Flexibility.
Solloway Mindfulness Survey (SMS) (Solloway & Fisher, 2007)	Solloway Mindfulness Survey is both a trait and state measure, developed to measure mindfulness from the perspective of mindfulness as a capacity to practice; a semi-changeable state with practice (state), but more trait-like in nature. This scale can be used for the purpose of tracking the progress of mindfulness students as they learn about mindfulness and begin their practice.
Kentucky Inventory of Mindfulness Skills (Baer et al., 2004).	This scale was developed to measure four mindfulness-related skills, as well as an overall tendency to be mindful during daily life. The four simple mindfulness skills include: Observing; Describing; Acting with awareness; and Accepting (or allowing) without judgment.
Toronto Mindfulness Scale (TMS) (Lau et al., 2006)	The Toronto scale is based on the conceptualization of mindfulness as an intentional, reflective style of introspection or self-observation, with the focus of attention being unrestricted.

The State Mindfulness Scale (SMS) (Tanay & Bernstein, 2013)	The SMS is intended to measure state mindfulness and conceptualizes mindfulness as a two-component construct, comprised of: Attention self-regulation, and an orientation to the present that involves curiosity, openness, and acceptance.
Philadelphia Mindfulness Scale (Cardaciotto et al., 2008)	This scale examines mindfulness as a bi-dimensional construct, composed of present-moment awareness and acceptance of the present state.
Acceptance & Action Questionnaire II (AAQ-II) (Bond et al., 2011)	Developed in order to establish an internally consistent measure of ACT. The measurement of acceptance on this scale is defined as the willingness to experience (i.e., not alter the form, frequency, or sensitivity of) unwanted private events, in the pursuit of one's values and goals.
Applied Mindfulness Process Scale (AMPS) (Li et al., 2016)	The AMPS quantifies how participants in mindfulness-based interventions use mindfulness practice when facing challenges in daily life. Three domains of applied mindfulness processes are measured by this scale: Decentering; Positive emotional regulation; and Negative emotional regulation.

the scale to those areas. Completing these scales at the beginning, middle, and end of intervention is a great way to track progress in being more mindful.

Assessment Summary

In sum, more research is needed in determining the utility and validity of mindfulness measures. Current best practice is to measure both the technique (e.g., level of mindful awareness) and the outcome (e.g., level of anxiety, depression, etc.). This allows you to assess both the effectiveness of a mindfulness intervention in facilitating improved mindfulness abilities, as well as improving emotional and/or behavioral well-being (Van Dam et al., 2010). The following case examples illustrate how the evaluation process could proceed in individual, group, and classroom-wide assessment, and in evaluating these practices with adult stakeholders.

Case Studies

Individual Youth: Matthew (he/him/his) is a 14-year-old presenting with anxiety. His school counselor, Mr. Davis, planned to treat him using mindfulness interventions; specifically, mindful breathing, use of the 5 senses technique, and focused meditation. Before beginning treatment, Mr. Davis administered a specific anxiety scale to assess his current level of general anxiety, in addition to administering the MAAS-A (Brown et al., 2011) to measure his current mindfulness levels. Mr. Davis chose the MAAS-A due to Matthew's age and also because higher levels of mindfulness, as measured on the MAAS-A, negatively correlate with self-reported stress and anxiety, while being positively correlated with happiness and healthy self-regulation. As predicted, Matthew initially rated himself as having clinically significant symptoms of anxiety and a low level of mindful awareness on the respective scales. Mr. Davis gave Matthew the scales to complete two more times over the span of working with him: once in the middle to monitor progress, and once at the end to assess any benefit from intervention. At the end of treatment, Matthew rated himself as having significantly fewer anxiety symptoms and increased mindfulness presence on the MAAS-A. Additionally, Matthew was attending school more regularly and had a small improvement in his grades.

   Small Group: Ms. Cosette, a school psychologist, plans to run a small (six youth, aged 16–17), 8-week mindfulness and acceptance-based group, as described in Chapter 5, for students referred to her for depression. Before the first group, Ms. Cosette decides to administer a self-report adolescent depression screener, along with the MTSA (West et al., 2007). The MTSA was chosen to use with this group, as it targets youths' ability to engage in healthy self-regulation and accept their life experiences. She found some variation across the youth, but overall, they scored within the moderate range of depressive symptoms; all had lower scores on the MTSA. Ms. Cosette administered both scales again mid-way through the group (week 4), as well as at the conclusion of the eight-week group. At the end of the group, the youth showed fewer depressive symptoms across group members and significantly higher scores in healthy self-regulation and acceptance practices on the MTSA. Because of this success, the school requested she run several other groups of teens using the same curriculum.

Classroom-Wide Intervention: Miss Sophie, a fifth-grade elementary teacher, decided to start a classroom-wide mindfulness program for her classroom of 10-year-olds. Practices in this program included breathwork, mindfulness, body scanning, acceptance, and cognitive defusion. Before she started the program, she administered a brief screener to her class. She chose the CAMM (Greco et al., 2011) because it is brief, only 10 items, appropriate for the age of her students, and measures present-moment awareness, as well as judgmental and nonaccepting responses to thoughts and feelings, which were processes directly targeted by the treatment components included in this program. Midway through the program, as well as at the conclusion of the 12-week mindfulness program, she administered the CAMM again. Following completion of the program, through both self-report on the CAMM and her behavioral observations, the majority of her classroom had achieved higher levels of present moment awareness and they appeared to be calmer and less reactive during the school day. Additionally, there were fewer disciplinary referrals after the intervention.

Adult Stakeholders: Mr. Bosco, the principal at the local middle school, saw that many of the teachers in his school were struggling with stress and symptoms of burnout. Mr. Bosco decided to hire a mindfulness consultant to conduct a day-long workshop on mindfulness education, focused on practical skills teachers could use immediately. In addition, he created a book club where his teachers all read the same book, *Get Out of Your Mind and Into Your Life: The New Acceptance and Commitment Therapy*, by Hayes and Smith (2005). The teachers met once a week after school for a month to discuss the chapters.

Before implementing the above interventions, Mr. Bosco measured teachers' current levels of burnout using the Maslach Burnout Inventory: Educators Survey (Maslach et al., 1996). He also used the AAQ-II (Bond et al., 2011) to measure current levels of acceptance and movement toward values-based goals and the Solloway Mindfulness Survey (Solloway & Fisher, 2007) to measure current state and trait mindful awareness in his teachers. After the workshop and the conclusion of the book club, Mr. Bosco readministered all scales, which showed improvement across all three measures. Mr. Boscoe decided to continue the mindfulness/ACT book club to help maintain these gains.

Conclusion

From working with youth suffering from anxiety or depression, to working with teachers on burnout prevention, mindfulness and acceptance practices have been shown to be invaluable tools for prevention, early intervention, and treatment. Mindfulness and acceptance practices are well-suited for use in an MTSS model in the schools, from individual and small group practice, to school-wide implementation, to working with adult stakeholders. However, given that the Western use of these practices is only a few decades old, especially when used with youth, it is imperative that well-designed research continue to assess these interventions to ensure we are using best practices for the youth, school-based professionals, and families we serve. Empirically evaluating how to adapt mindfulness practices with various populations should also occur.

References

Baer, R. A., Smith, G. T., & Allen, K. B. (2004). Assessment of mindfulness by self-report: The Kentucky inventory of mindfulness skills. *Assessment, 11*(3), 191–206.

Baer, R. A., Smith, G. T., Hopkins, J., Krietemeyer, J., & Toney, L. (2006). Using self-report assessment methods to explore facets of mindfulness. *Assessment, 13*(1), 27–45.

Bond, F. W., Hayes, S. C., Baer, R. A., Carpenter, K. M., Guenole, N., Orcutt, H. K., Waltz, T., & Zettle, R. D. (2011). Preliminary psychometric properties of the acceptance and action questionnaire – II: A revised measure of psychological flexibility and experiential avoidance. *Behavior Therapy, 42*, 676–688.

Brown, K. W., & Ryan, R. M. (2003). The benefits of being present: Mindfulness and its role in psychological well-being. *Journal of Personality and Social Psychology, 84*(4), 822–848.

Brown, K. W., West, A. M., Loverich, T. M., & Biegel, G. M. (2011). Assessing adolescent mindfulness: Validation of an adapted Mindful Attention Awareness Scale in adolescent normative and psychiatric populations. *Psychological Assessment, 23*(4), 1023–1033.

Cardaciotto, L., Herbert, J. D., Forman, E. M., Moitra, E., & Farrow, V. (2008). The assessment of present-moment awareness and acceptance: The Philadelphia Mindfulness Scale. *Assessment, 15*(2), 204–223.

de Bruin, E. I., Zijlstra, B. J., & Bögels, S. M. (2014). The meaning of mindfulness in children and adolescents: Further validation of the Child and Adolescent Mindfulness Measure (CAMM) in two independent samples from the Netherlands. *Mindfulness, 5*(4), 422–430.

de Bruin, E. I., Zijlstra, B. J. H., van de Weijer-Bergsma, E., & Bögels, S. M. (2011). The mindful attention awareness scale for adolescents (MAAS-A): Psychometric properties in a Dutch sample. *Mindfulness, 2*(3), 201–211.

Feldman, G., Hayes, A., Kumar, S., Greeson, J., & Laurenceau, J.-P. (2007). Mindfulness and emotion regulation: The development and initial validation of the Cognitive and Affective Mindfulness Scale-Revised (CMS-R). *Journal of Psychopathology and Behavioral Assessment, 29*(3), 177–190.

Greco, L. A., Baer, R. A., & Smith, G. T. (2011). Assessing mindfulness in children and adolescents: Development and validation of the Child and Adolescent Mindfulness Measure (CAMM). *Psychological Assessment, 23*(3), 606–614.

Guerra, J., García-Gómez, M., Turanzas, J., Cordón, J., Suárez-Jurado, C., & Mestre, J. (2019). A brief Spanish version of the child and adolescent mindfulness\ measure (CAMM): A dispositional mindfulness measure. *International Journal of Environmental Research and Public Health, 16*(8), 1355.

Hayes, S. C., & Smith, S. (2005). *Get out of your mind and into your life: The new acceptance and commitment therapy.* New Harbinger Publications.

Kuby, A. K., McLean, N., & Allen, K. (2015). Validation of the child and adolescent mindfulness measure (CAMM) with non-clinical adolescents. *Mindfulness, 6*(6), 1448–1455.

Lau, M. A., Bishop, S. R., Segal, Z. V., Buis, T., Anderson, N. D., Carlson, L., Shapiro, S., Carmody, J., Abbey, S., & Devins, G. (2006). The Toronto mindfulness scale: Development and validation. *Journal of Clinical Psychology, 62*(12), 1445–1467.

Li, M. J., Black, D. S., & Garland, E. L. (2016). The Applied Mindfulness Process Scale (AMPS): A process measure for evaluating mindfulness-based interventions. *Personality and Individual Differences, 93*, 6–15.

Manuel, J. A., Somohano, V. C., & Bowen, S. (2017). Mindfulness practice and its relationship to the five-facet mindfulness questionnaire. *Mindfulness, 8*(2), 361–367.

Maslach, C., Jackson, S., & Leiter, M. (1996). *The Maslach Burnout Inventory-Test Manual.* Library of Congress.

Pirson, M., Langer, E., Bodner, T., & Zilcha-Mano, S. (2012). The development and validation of the Langer Mindfulness Scale – enabling a socio-cognitive perspective of mindfulness in organizational contexts. *Fordham University Schools of Business Research Paper.*

Ristallo, A., Schweiger, M., Oppo, A., Pergolizzi, F., Presti, G., & Moderato, P. (2016). Misurare la mindfulness in età evolutiva: Proprietà psicometriche e struttura fattoriale della versione italiana della Child and Adolescent Mindfulness Measure (I-CAMM) [Measuring child and adolescent mindfulness: Psychometric properties and factorial structure of the Italian version of the Child and Adolescent Mindfulness Measure (I-CAMM)]. *Psicoterapia Cognitiva e Comportamentale, 22*(3), 297–315.

Solloway, S. G., & Fisher, W. P., Jr. (2007). Mindfulness in measurement: Reconsidering the measurable in mindfulness practice. *International Journal of Transpersonal Studies, 26*, 58–81.

Sünbül, Z. A. (2018). Psychometric evaluation of child and adolescent mindfulness measure (CAMM) with a Turkish sample. *International Journal of Education and Psychological Research, 7*, 56–59.

Tanay, G., & Bernstein, A. (2013). State Mindfulness Scale (SMS): Development and initial validation. *Psychological Assessment, 25*(4), 1286–1299.

Van Dam, N. T., Earleywine, M., & Borders, A. (2010). Measuring mindfulness? An item response theory analysis of the mindful attention awareness scale. *Personality and Individual Differences, 49*(7), 805–810.

Walach, H., Buchheld, N., Buttenmüller, V., Kleinknecht, N., & Schmidt, S. (2006). Measuring mindfulness – The Freiburg Mindfulness Inventory (FMI). *Personality and Individual Differences, 40*(8), 1543–1555.

West, A. M. (2008). Mindfulness and well-being in adolescence: An exploration of four mindfulness measures with an adolescent sample. *Dissertation Abstracts International: Section B: The Sciences and Engineering, 69*(5-B), 3283.

West, A. M., Sbraga, T. P., & Poole, D. A. (2007). *Measuring mindfulness in youth: Development of the Mindful Thinking and Action Scale for Adolescents* [Unpublished manuscript]. Central Michigan University.

Index